Mnemonics, Rhetoric and Poetics for Medics

COVER

A variation on a famous Persian miniature etching of Avicenna (980-1037). Avicenna was a brilliant physician well known for his vast memory (by age ten he knew the Koran by heart). He also had a reputation of being a drunkard and a wanderer. His greatest achievement was his Canon of Medicine, a verbose textbook, in which he explains controversial subjects such as why breasts don't grow on the belly and why calves are not on the front of the legs.

Mnemonics, Rhetoric and Poetics for Medics

Knowledge worth spewing not requiring emetics

Robert L. Bloomfield, M.D.
Instructor, Department of Medicine
Bowman Gray School of Medicine
Wake Forest University
Winston-Salem, N.C.

E. Ted Chandler, M.D.
Associate Professor
Department of Medicine
Bowman Gray School of Medicine
Wake Forest University
Winston-Salem, N.C.

Also by E. Ted Chandler, M.D.
How To Have Good Health

Inquiries should be addressed to
Harbinger Press
Box 17201
Winston-Salem, N.C. 27106

Printed and bound by Hunter Publishing Company, Winston-Salem, N.C.
27103

Library of Congress Catalogue Number 82-81637

ISBN 0-89459-171-1

To
Carolyn, Adam, Fran, Lynn and Steve

Acknowledgements:

In lieu of free lunches we acknowledge the gracious help of Vernon Foster, Geraldine Zurek, Cecilia Hartsoe, Jeff Ausband, Jill Kirkpatrick, Ginny Thomas, Mary Ingalls for her original art work and Carolyn Pedley for her original art.

Table of Contents

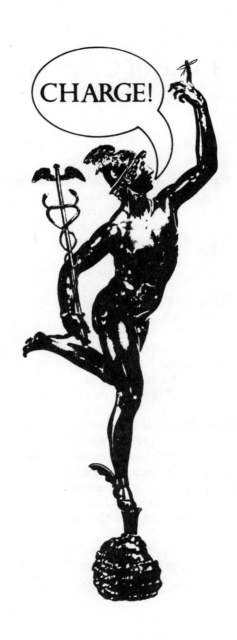

Preface

"Knowledge may be an encumbrance as well as a help. Many men know more than they are able to wield. There is a point . . . in the acquisition of knowledge . . . beyond which if more be acquired, the whole mass becomes useless to its possessor."

— Latham

"A small overweight of knowledge is often a sore impediment to the movements of common sense."

— Latham

This book is written for all those who, in the daily practice of medicine, are faced with the limitations of their memory and the finiteness of their minds. Delving into the logical science of general medicine necessitates a certain amount of leisure time, whereas the responsibilities of clinical practice seem to be of never ending emergence. Because of this there is a great benefit to be found in simplified means of remembering medical knowledge; methods which allow our barraged Betz cells to take a breather; ways to let them lean back on our limbic system so that our convolutions can convalesce.

Those late night admissions or early morning emergency room visits are the true tests of our recall facilities. Like the overhead surgical lamp, they reveal too clearly the wrinkles and gaps in our informational facade. The larger gaps obviously require further study and experience for filler, but it is safe and expedient to seal the smaller spaces with the help of maxims, mnemonics and aphorisms.

In those wee hours when we are functioning primarily on our reptilian brains, mnemonics become particularly useful, for they appeal to our perceptions more than to our logic. They represent a more convenient arrangement for retrieval of those facts we once thought we knew so well. They politely avoid the overrefinement which tends to permeate research papers and medical treatises. At their best they neatly "wrap up wisdom in a witticism."

There are several notes of caution to keep in mind, however. One is that oversimplification is a common pitfall of many memory devices. In a study on the use of these methods, Bursztajn and Hamm have adeptly pointed out the limited utility of rigid maxims (the mechanistic paradigms) and the greater faith which can be placed in maxims that start with probabilities, therefore articulating more complex and flexible aphorisms (the probabilistic paradigm.)

Another shortcoming of mnemonics, though not peculiar to them, is overgeneralization and the false sense of security in diagnostic pursuit it may create. The eagerness to come to conclusions is a major stumbling block to the collection of clinical "facts." As Latham put it "there is no such thing as turning practical medicine into a well told tale."

With these things kept in proper perspective, we hope our readers will digest these medical tidbits with pleasure and amusement. We trust they will impart some useful information and impress it on the mind in a form that will make it readily accessible over and over again. May the time it saves you fortifying your memories be spent improving your clinical judgement for which there is no substitute.

R.L.B.
E.T.C.

Chapter I

Mnemonics

Aphorisms, Acronyms, Acrostics, Abecedarius and Alliteration

"The writer of text books should have a ready imagination and he should understand the child's mind."

C. H. Mayo

The main thrust of this book is to provide several approaches to remembering medical knowledge. These are, in the authors' opinion, the best approaches. Imprinting material into long term memory is best accomplished by organizing information in accordance with the inherent characteristics of the information itself. As an example, let's consider the differential diagnosis of expiratory splitting and paradoxical splitting of the second heart sound. In contrast to fixed splitting, which occurs almost exclusively in those conditions that cause right ventricular overload or pulmonary hypertension (atrial septal defects, ventricular septal defects, massive or chronic pulmonary embolism and congestive heart failure), paradoxical splitting occurs in those processes which affect conduction, contraction or blood flow of the left side of the heart (aortic stenosis, aortic regurgitation, idiopathic hypertrophic subaortic stenosis, supra or subvalvular aortic stenosis, systemic hypertension, left bundle branch block and left sided myocardial infarction). Expiratory splitting occurs in those processes which predominantly affect contraction, conduction or blood flow of the right side of the heart (pulmonic stenosis, pulmonic valve regurgitation, pulmonary hypertension, atrial septal defects, ventricular septal defects, right bundle branch block, "right sided" myocardial infarction and idiopathic dilatation of the pulmonary artery).

This categorization, though slightly over generalized, makes

1

physiologic sense and serves as a simplified way of recalling these auscultatory findings. Unfortunately, this physiologic and more deductive method of recollection is not usually feasible with regard to long and complex lists of differential diagnoses such as these.

The alternatives are methods which impose a more contrived system of organization on the information to be memorized; such techniques as mediation, imagery and mnemonics have been well outlined by Cermak. These methods are especially powerful and useful for remembering lists of items that do not neatly fit into our established network of knowledge.

Mnemonics, an all inclusive term to describe all these techniques, are often quite arbitrary in the means of composition. However, there is no reason why we cannot create them in forms which make them bearers of imagery, thus providing additional information beyond a mere list of items. They then become a link to related knowledge, serve as a springboard to other memories and therefore, become more useful and recallable.

In the past, medical mnemonics have taken a relatively simple form — the acrostic or acronym. For our purposes, the acrostic can be defined as a set of initial letters from a group of words which, when written in a particular order, form a word, phrase or abbreviation. The word V-I-N-D-I-C-A-T-E and the phrase M-A-N-I-A-C   T-V, for example, have each been used as acronyms for the general approach to the varied causes of any particular set of symptoms and signs.

Vindicate:
<u>V</u>ascular causes
<u>I</u>nflammatory or infectious disease
<u>N</u>eoplastic disorders
<u>D</u>egenerative or deficiency states
<u>I</u>ntoxication
<u>C</u>ongenital causes
<u>A</u>utoimmune or allergic disease
<u>T</u>rauma
<u>E</u>ndocrine (including metabolic) disorders.

Maniac — TV:

<u>M</u>etabolic disease
<u>A</u>natomic disorder
<u>N</u>eoplastic disease
<u>I</u>nfectious disease
<u>A</u>llergic disorder
<u>C</u>ollagen vascular disease
<u>T</u>rauma
<u>V</u>ascular disease.

Anatomy students who have dissected the inguinal region of a cadaver in the line of course work have heard the acronym N-A-V-E-L, which represents the inguinal structures passing from lateral to medial side:

<u>N</u>erve
<u>A</u>rtery
<u>V</u>ein
<u>E</u>mpty space
<u>L</u>ymphatic

By constructing a word-picture, these previous examples aid our recall ability because they become a part of our permanent memory bank. It is preferable to design acronyms so that they spell out words which are in some respect related to the intended concept. In these cases, the bond between the mnemonic device and the memorized material is strengthened, thus easing the process in which the whole pattern is imprinted in the memory. Several examples follow:

The muscles of mastication:
Mnemonic: B-I-T-E-M

<u>B</u>uccinator — (from the Latin word for trumpeter) lines the cheek and with the help of the tongue helps to keep food poised between the molars.

<u>I</u>nternal pterygoid — (same as medial pterygoid) originates from the medial pterygoid plate and inserts on the ramus of the mandible. Its general shape, direction and actions are similar to the masseter.

<u>T</u>emporalis — a powerful biting muscle fanning out from the side

of the cranium and inserting on the coronoid process of the mandible.

External pterygoid — (same as lateral pterygoid) lies in a horizontal plane originating from the lateral pterygoid plate and inserting near the mandibular joint. Its actions protrude the jaw and, with the opposite external pterygoid produce side to side motion.

Masseter — (from the Greek word for chewer) is a powerful rectangular muscle stretching from the zygomatic arch to the mandibular angle.

Now consider this acrostic for the major neurotransmitters:
Mnemonic: S-E-N-D

Serotonin — a neurotransmitter whose precise function is not yet completely clear, but with a known capacity to cause smooth muscle contraction in the blood vessels and gut. It has been hypothesized to play a role in the initial phase of migraine headache. In carcinoid, serotonin plays a role in producing the intestinal hypermotility associated with the syndrome. It is not, however, responsible for the flush which may be due to bradykinin or catecholamines.

Epinephrine — the main storage form of neurotransmitter found in the adrenal medulla, release of which is provoked by the four H's (the Four H club) — hypoxia, hemorrhagic hypotension, hard work and hypoglycemia. A proportion of epinephrine is derived by N-methylation of . . .

Norepinephrine — like epinephrine, causes physiologic responses preparing the organism for "fight or flight" (rapid, deep respiration, constriction of cutaneous and renal vessels, inotropic and chronotropic cardiac effect). Unlike epinephrine it has a predominantly vasoconstrictor effect and its release is not provoked by hypoglycemia. Its biosynthetic precursor is . . .

Dopamine — stimulates beta-adrenergic receptors causing both inotropic and chronotropic effects on the heart and producing renal and mesenteric vasodilatation. When administered as intravenous medication in doses above 10 ug/kg/min, alpha

4

adrenergic effects (vasoconstriction) tend to predominate. Dopamine causes less of an increase in arterial pressure and more of an increase in cardiac output than norepinephrine.

An onomatopoetic mnemonic is this one for aid in the evaluation of traumatic emergencies:
Mnemonic: C-R-A-S-H   P-L-A-N

Cardiac — assessing the need for circulatory support.

Respiratory — establishing a clear airway and adequate ventilation.

Abdominal — in nonpenetrating wounds evidence of injury may not be manifest for several hours. In penetrating injuries, if peritoneal penetration is ruled out, local treatment is in order. Otherwise, the need for nasogastric tube, rectal exam, bladder catheter and upright and supine x-rays should be assessed.

Spine — in the unconscious patient, maintaining a high index of suspicion for spinal injury is warranted. Moving the patient en bloc to avoid further injury is essential. Palpate from head to coccyx in search of malalignment or reflex withdrawal to painful stimulus. Absent deep tendon reflexes or withdrawal responses suggest spinal shock. See Table I in the appendix (pp. 210) for testing motor and sensory levels.

Head — perform a quick but thorough neurological exam with special attention to frequent assessment of the state of consciousness, pupillary size and reactivity, eye movements, deep tendon reflexes, motor function, and ear or nasal bleeding.

Pelvis — fractures of the bony pelvis can cause bladder perforation or urethral injuries. Treatment of bladder perforation is always emergent, requiring exploration, drainage of the perivesical space and suprapubic cystostomy. In urethral injuries, the site of disruption is confirmed by retrograde urethrogram and suprapubic cystostomy is employed to facilitate healing.

Limbs — evaluate for fractures, contusions, ligamentous tears and occult damage to . . .

<u>A</u>rteries and
<u>N</u>erves.

These last acrostics show a closer correspondence to their subject matter than the initial examples and, for this reason, we feel they are more perfect in form, more graceful and a tad more "poetic." Later we'll present some mnemonics which take further advantage of this "poetic" aspect, (though admittedly they show little resemblance to any of Homer's works).

Epi-acronyms

One adaption of the acrostic technique, in which the initial letters of the words in a phase serve as an alphabetic cue to recollect some group of items, is represented by the term epi-acronym.

The classic example of this is the well-known metered rhyme to help recall the nomenclature for the twelve cranial nerves:

ON-OLD-OLYMPIC-TOWERING-TOPS
A-FIN-AND-GERMAN-VIEWED-SOME-HOPS

<u>On</u>-olfactory (I) — the delicate fibers of the first cranial nerves pass through the cribriform plate, where they are easily damaged by fractures, meningeal disorders, or nasal mucosal disease. Each nostril is tested separately with a non-irritating substance (vanilla, coffee, tobacco). Pungent substances cause trigeminal stimulation.

<u>Old</u>-optic (II) — optic nerve injury can be secondary to a variety of disorders including trauma, toxins, systemic disease such as diabetes, syphilis, T.B., leukemia, giant cell arteritis, demyelinating diseases, tumors, glaucoma, thrombosis of associated blood vessels or increased intracranial pressure of any cause. Visual field testing, visual acuity, and funduscopic exam are the modes of evaluation.

<u>Olympic</u>-oculomotor (III) — this nerve supplies five extrinsic eye muscles; medial rectus, superior rectus, inferior rectus, inferior oblique, and levator palpebrae. The picture of complete third nerve palsy includes ptosis, deviation of the eyeball outward and slightly downward, and pupillary dilatation with

loss of light reaction and accomodation. The most frequent cause is an aneurysm in the circle of Willis.

Towering-trochlear (IV) — the motor nerve to the superior oblique muscle runs a roundabout course passing by the superior cerebellar and cerebral peduncles, the posterior clinoid process and through the cavernous sinus and superior orbital fissure. Lesions of the nerve cause an inability to gaze downward and outward with the affected eye. The patient attempts to compensate by tilting the head to the opposite shoulder.

Tops-trigeminal (V) — this is the tops in cranial nerves; that is, the largest one. It provides sensation to the superficial and deep structures of the face and motor innervation to the muscles of mastication (see B-I-T-E-M p. 3) Additionally, it carries the fibers responsible for both corneal and sneezing reflexes. Irritation of the sensory portion causes tic douloureux.

A-abducens (VI) — sixth nerve injury causes lateral rectus ocular muscle paralysis, producing inward deviation of the affected eye. Paralysis of lateral gaze occurs when the sixth nerve nucleus in the brainstem is damaged. In this case, intactness of the medial rectus of the unaffected opposite eye can be demonstrated by testing for convergence.

Fin-facial (VII) — a complex nerve carrying motor sensory and autonomic signals, the seventh nerve has two main divisions. The first, nervus intermedius, carries taste sensation from the anterior two-thirds of the tongue and fibers which innervate salivary and lacrimal glands. The motor division supplies the facial muscles. Lesions occurring in the motor cortex, prior to the facial nerve nucleus in the brainstem (upper motor neuron), partially spare forehead and upper eyelid muscles.

And-acoustic (VIII) — this nerve is composed of two functionally separate parts, the cochlear and vestibular nerves. Involvement of the former division causes hearing loss and tinnitus. Vestibular disorders cause vertigo and nystagmus. (see mnemonic for differential diagnosis of vertigo p. 178)

German-glossopharyngeal (IX) — the ninth nerve carries sensory information from the upper pharynx and taste sensation from the posterior third of the tongue. An isolated lesion is rare and causes little in the way of dysfunction unless painful neuralgia is associated. A gag reflex demonstrates that the nerve is intact.

Viewed-vagus (X) — the vagal fibers from the nucleus ambiguous supply the muscles of the pharynx and larynx. This is easy to remember since the larynx has always been the major source of all ambiguity. The dorsal motor nucleus sends autonomic fibers to the heart, lungs, esophagus and stomach. The examiner tests the vagus along with the ninth nerve, looking for uvula deviation, elevation of the larynx with swallowing or hoarseness.

Some-spinal accessory (XI) — the eleventh nerve innervates the trapezius and sternocleidomastoid, which are easily tested by having the patient shrug his shoulders and rotate his head against resistance.

Hops-hypoglossal (XII) — the motor nerve to the tongue can be affected by all those processes which affect the nuclei of the tenth and eleventh nerves; amyotrophic lateral sclerosis, syringobulbia, demyelinating diseases or tumors. Unilateral paralysis causes deviation toward the weak side; bilateral paralysis produces difficulty with eating and lingual speech (e.g. round the rugged rock the ragged rascal ran).

Those individuals with a proclivity for the more ribald devices might prefer the mnemonic Oh-Oh-Oh-To-Touch-And-Feel-A-Girl's-Vagina,-So-Heavenly for the cranial nerves. We personally prefer the former example, not only because it displays better taste (we love hops), but also because it is a little less distracting.

Another well-known epi-acronym is Oh.-P.-T.-Barnum-Loves-The-Kids, representing neoplasms which are prone to metastasize to bone. However, the following alternative is much neater in its approach and serves the same purpose better.

Mnemonic: KINDS-OF-TUMORS
  LEAPING-PROMPTLY-TO-BONE

Kinds (kidney) — in adults, the most common renal neoplasm is the hypernephroma. Half the cases will present with hematuria, flank pain or an abdominal mass. The tumor is noted for its relative radioresistance and its association with paraneoplastic syndromes.

Of (ovary) — eighty five percent of ovarian cancers arise from the surface of the ovary (germinal epithelium). The remainder originate from either ovarian stroma (granulosa theca cell tumor, arrhenoblastoma) or from the ovum itself. In premenopausal women an adnexal mass less than 6 cm. is usually a physiologic cyst and can be observed for several weeks. The same finding in a postmenopausal woman demands immediate definitive diagnosis.

Tumors (testis) — testicular cancer is the most frequent tumor found in young males. The acronym T-E-S-T-I-C stands for the most common varieties; (**T**eratocarcinoma, **E**mbryonal carcinoma, **S**eminoma, **T**eratoma, **I**nterstitial **C**ell tumor). The firm, painless testicular mass must be differentiated from chronic tuberculous or gonorrheal epididymitis, hydroceles and spermatoceles.

Leaping (lung) — the approach to the diagnosis and staging of lung cancer starts with the noninvasive procedures such as sputum cytologies, estimation of nodule doubling time (usually 10-400 days in malignant diseases) and biopsies of palpable scalene nodes. For further evaluation, the sites and number of lesions and general health of the patient will help determine the best approach.

Promptly (prostate) — a prevalent disease with a widely variable course, prostatic cancer presents in twenty percent of cases with symptoms due to metastatic disease (especially bone pain). Rectal examination, the most practical means of detection, only identifies ten percent of cases.

To (thyroid) — the most common forms of thyroid carcinoma are designated papillary and follicular. A mixed type of these two varieties is relatively common. The follicular elements are responsible for the early hematogenous dissemination to bone and lung. Pure papillary carcinoma tends toward slow growth and spreads to local lymph nodes.

Bone (breast) — unusual in its pattern of metastatic involvement, distant lesions may develop many years after diagnosis and apparently successful treatment. However, in patients with a mass less than five cm. without lymph node involvement, the ten year survival rate is seventy percent. With lymph node spread the survival rate drops to ten to twenty percent.

Cue words such as these short cut the memory process since the statement itself reveals the material that is to be remembered. The previous examples all required a second transposition in recalling what the sentence stood for.

Another popular epi-acronym is this one for the carpal bones: NEVER-LOWER-TILLEY'S-PANTS,-MAMMA-MIGHT-COME-HOME.

Never (navicular) also called scaphoid.
Lower (lunate).
Tilley's (triquetrum).
Pants (pisiform).
Mamma (greater multangular) also called trapezium.
Might (lesser multangular) also called trapezoid.
Come (capitate).
Home (hamate).

We might footnote that one with this mnemonic phrase for the tarsal bones: CONNIE-COULDN'T-COUNT-CUBES NEVER-TACKLED-CALCULUS.*

Connie (1st cuneiform).
Couldn't (2nd cuneiform).
Count (3rd cuneiform).
Cubes (cuboid).
Never (navicular).
Tackled (talus).
Calculus (calcaneus).

This epi-acronym is superior to its predecessor in that each clue word approximates phonetically the word we are attempting to retrieve. The longer the list of items, the more appropriate it is to instill this quality in the phrase. Constructing such a mnemonic for a longer, more challenging list of things often happily surprises the composer and memorizer. They discover that the complex phrases may be the easiest to remember because there are more cue words to provide the opportunity for combining descriptive terms. These, in turn, create vivid imagery which more than compensates for the increased number of items.

Examples: Coumadin drug interactions in Vivo.
Drugs that Potentiate Coumadin

Mnemonic:　　　NORTON-INDULGED-QUINN'S-PROPER-PHILADELPHIAN-AUNTS-SOLICITOUSLY.
ALAS-ANNA-CLOEY-CLARA and GLUE SNIFFING-MIFFY-SIMULTANEOUSLY-SUFFERED-SINFUL-AUNTABUSE.*

Norton (Nortriptyline)
　　Mechanism: unknown.

Indulged (Indomethacin)
　　Mechanism: impairs platelet function.

Quinn's (Quinine, Quinidine)
　　Mechanism: ? displacement from binding sites.
　　　　　　? platelet antibody formation.

Proper (Propylthiouracil)
　　Mechanism: unknown.

Philadelphian (Phenylbutazone)
　　Mechanism: displacement from binding sites.

Aunts (Antibiotics; Sulfonamides and Chloramphenicol)
　　Mechanism: displacement from binding sites and inhibition of microsomal enzymes, respectively.

Solicitously (Salicylates)
　　Mechanism: impairs platelet function.

Alas (Allopurinol)
　　Mechanism: inhibits microsomal enzymes.

Anna (Anabolic steroids)
　　Mechanism: unknown.

Cloey (Clofibrate)
　　Mechanism: displacement from binding sites.

Clara (Chloral hydrate)
Mechanism: displacement from binding sites.

Gluesniffing (Glucagon)
Mechanism: ? increased catabolism of clotting factors.

Miffy (Mefenamic acid) — related to salicylates
Mechanism: impairs platelet function.

Simultaneously (Cimetidine)
Mechanism: ? displacement from binding sites.

Suffered (Sulfinpyrazone) — related to phenylbutazone
Mechanism: impairs platelet function.

Sinful (Synthroid and other thyroid medications)
Mechanism: increased catabolism of clotting factors.

Auntabuse (Antabuse-Disulfiram)
Mechanism: inhibition of microsomal enzymes.

Drugs that Inhibit Coumadin
Mnemonic:
BARBARA'S-COLOSSAL-GLUTEUS MAXIMAE
REVAMP-GRIZZLED-ESTABLISHMENTARIANS*

Barbara's (Barbiturates)
Mechanism: induction of microsomal enzymes.

Colossal (Cholestyramine)
Mechanism: decreased anticoagulant absorption.

Gluteus maximae (Glutethimide)
Mechanism: induction of microsomal enzymes.

Revamp (Rifampin)
Mechanism: induction of microsomal enzymes.

Grizzled (Griseofulvin)
Mechanism: induction of microsomal enzymes.

Establishmentarians (Estrogen preparations — eg. oral contraceptives)
Mechanism: increased synthesis or activity of some clotting factors.

The main principles which govern the composition of epiacronyms such as these are vivid imagery, rhyme and homonyms.

Additionally, the act of composition in itself will do much to indelibly etch items into our memory.

Alliteration and an Ally, Abecedarius.

Our final examples of mean and simple methods for maximizing medical maxim memorization is (can you guess?) that rhetorical device in which one repeats the same sound in sequential words: alliteration. Consider, for example, some symptoms and signs of Addison's disease.

The A's of Addison's Disease

Asthenia — general debilitation and loss of libido are cardinal early symptoms. The reasons for drowsiness, headache, confusion and the occasional occurrence of papilledema and increased intracranial pressure are unexplained.

Anorexia — will lead to a very attenuated individual. It occurs in up to ninety percent of patients.

Abdominal pain — occurs in nearly a third of patients. It is usually ill defined, but may imitate an acute abdomen. Other common gastrointestinal symptoms include nausea, vomiting and diarrhea.

Anxiety.

Arterial hypotension — with accentuation of postural changes is a frequent finding and may lead to syncope. As with the symptoms listed above it is common to both primary and secondary adrenal apoplexy.

Aches (muscle cramps) — are due to salt wastage. Salt craving is seen in primary but not secondary adrenal insufficiency. Ascending paralysis associated with hyperkalemia is an unusual manifestation of primary disease.

Axillary, **A**nal and **A**reolar pigmentation (as well as pigmentation of palmar creases, scars, knuckles, knees and buccal mucosa) — occurs in ninety eight percent of patients with primary disease and essentially none of those with the secondary form. Hyperpigmentation, due to increased amounts of MSH and ACTH, can be seen in conjunction with cancers causing Cushing's syndrome. (For differential diagnosis of hyperpigmentation see p. 150)

Aldosterone deficiency in Addison's disease — causes renal loss of sodium with resultant hyponatremia. Aldosterone deficiency along with associated acidosis are the major factors contributing to the hyperkalemia seen in this disorder.

ACTH testing with alpha-1-24-adrenocorticotropin (cortrosyn) assays adrenal reserve and aids in differentiating between primary and secondary forms. (See appendix p. 215)

Additionally, seventy-five percent of cases of adrenal apoplexy are of autoimmune origin with circulating antibodies to adrenal cell antigens. Associated with Addison's are atrophic gastritis and pernicious anemia.

Also attributed to Thomas Addison is the artful description of Vitamin B_{12} deficiency which he called "idiopathic anemia." The causes of this previously fatal disease are catagorized in the following alliterative mnemonic.

The I's of Vitamin B_{12} Deficiency*

Intrinsic factor deficiency — (pernicious anemia, gastrectomy, congenital absence) Intrinsic factor (IF) is a glycoprotein secreted by parietal cells in the stomach which forms a complex with the Vitamin B_{12} from ingested food.

Ileal inflammation or resection — (Whipples disease, tropical sprue, nontropical sprue, regional enteritis) In the distal ileum, specific mucosal receptors bind the Vitamin B_{12}-IF complex and the vitamin is transferred across the mucosa into the circulation.

Infected intestine — (bacterial overgrowth in strictures and blind loops) Large amounts of bacteria colonizing the small intestine compete for the Vitamin B_{12} . A similar situation occurs in . . .

Infestation of the intestine with tapeworm (diphylobothrium latum) most often seen in Finland.

Rare causes include:

Inadequate intake — (vegetarians)

Immerslund's syndrome — a selective congenital defect in intestinal absorption of B_{12} which is also associated with proteinuria.

Closely related to alliteration is abecedarius. (This is not to be confused with abracadabra, the cabalistic charm concocted from the initials of the words for Father-Ab, Son-Ben, and Holy Spirit — Ruach Acadseh, and used as an ancient antidote against ague and other ailments.) (See appendix p. 216)

Abecedarius refers to the method of using each successive letter of the alphabet as the initial part of a group of words or stanzas. For instance:

The ABC's of Lead Poisoning

A — Anemia is generally mild. Pallor is more than would be expected for the degree of anemia and is thought to be due to arteriolar constriction. The mechanism of the anemia is probably a combination of erythrocyte fragility and a maturation defect. The peripheral blood film reveals numerous red cells with . . .

B — Basophilic stippling — The striking coarse stippling which consists of RNA, iron and mitochondria can also occur in megaloblastic anemia. Fine stippling occurs in any situation where there is increased red blood cell production.

C — Colic — The abdominal pain of lead toxicity is poorly localized and is accompanied by rigid muscular spasm of the abdominal wall. Fever and leukocytosis are notably absent and the pain is unresponsive to morphine. Calcium, however, effectively relieves the pain in a short time.

D — Dementia — In a demented adult who has, in the past years, worked with solder, batteries, paints or illicit distilleries, one should consider lead poisoning as a prime possibility.

E — Encephalopathy, on the other hand, occurs almost exclusively in children. Manifestations include ataxia, vomiting and lethargy which can progress rapidly to seizures and coma. Mortality is high and, in those who survive, a full twenty-five percent will have severe permanent brain damage.

F — Foot drop (or wrist drop) can occur in the absence of other symptoms and is characteristic of peripheral lead neuropathy. It usually affects the nerves supplying the muscle groups used most by the affected individual.

G — Gingival pigmentation — The gum margin may be darkened in a linear fashion by lead sulfide. It is a rare finding in children and will be absent in edentulous patients.

The abecedarius is one of the oldest known memory aids. The lengthy 119th psalm in the Old Testament is constructed in this form, and attests to the fact that even the greatest teachers need an occasional mnemonic to stimulate their minds and perhaps, also, their students.

The chapters which follow contain other schemes for improving recall as well as further examples of the simple devices outlined in this chapter. Our own original mnemonics have been marked with an asterisk. Where appropriate, both traditional and original mnemonics have been adorned with vignettes or illustrations which are intended to frame these imperfect poems and make them more portable.

CHAPTER 2

Memory — An Overview

"There are people who are born with extraordinary memories (idiot savants among them), and there are people who train their memories into a condition of extraordinariness (fellows who have memorized the Manhattan telephone directory or can name twenty-seven films in which Akim Tamiroff did not play a character named Mohammed), but memory at its most impressive is that of the truly superior mind, whose memory is owed to study, to thoughtfulness, and to the integration of all the forces of intellection . . . And so it has seemed to me among the few powerful scholars I have known. They have only to press the button of memory to call up the most wondrous network of associations. Their suitcases have a great deal more in them because they are so much more intelligently packed. Next to them I think of myself as a man in a crowded railway station, schlepping three shopping bags, out of which obtrude bits of tissue, comic books, soiled linen. A cigarette is perched behind my ear, even though I do not smoke; and my raincoat pockets are stuffed with sheet music and old socks. Such at any rate is the self-view of one man whose memory is giving him difficulty."

Aristides

Enhancement of the memory is an art and a skill. Its origins lie deep in antiquity, meticulously unearthed by renaissance scholars and experimental psychologists who have searched for the truth of its nature and even yet find it elusive.

The human soul was often believed by the medieval philosophers, and Greek philosophers before them, to be linked externally to the five senses and internally to the imagination and memory. Thus Plato sensed the soul's recollection of ideas as the most truly important knowledge.

In the ancient world stone tablets were immobile and papyrus scarce. The dearth of printed matter made memory imperative for all learning, and the subject of memory was part of the more general study of rhetoric. Consider how impressive was the mental gymnastic of Simonides of Ceos in the sixth century B.C., when he identified, by their positions at the table, over one hundred guests who were crushed beneath a building that collapsed just as Simonides left the banquet hall. Seneca, famous for his memory, was said to have been able to repeat two thousand names in the order in which they were given to him. Augustine, himself a teacher of rhetoric, speaks of a friend named one Simplicus who was supposed to have been able to recite all of Vergil backward. Saint Thomas Aquinas not only had a prodigious memory, but was, in addition, a great authority on the subject. The most famous classical work on rhetoric is a how-to-do-it volume entitled *Ad Herennium* (c 86-82 B.C.) by an author who for some centuries was thought to be Tullius, but whose true name, according to Professor Frances A. Yates, is now acknowledged to be lost to history. Thus, the first of endless ironies on this matter of memory — forgotten is the author of the world's most influential book on the subject. Today's medical scholars, no less than those scholars of every genre in preceding generations, will find that the importance of memory can scarcely be overstated.

The number of new bits of exclusively medical knowledge which must be incorporated into the synaptic maze of a thinking doctor has been stated in a medical publication, but, for the life of me, I can't remember the number or where I read it. I can remember that it exceeded the number of moves that a chess player must learn in order to become a master. That's just the beginning. Consider the number of times that batch of knowledge is turned over, patched, renewed or completely refurbished throughout a lifetime devoted to medicine. As the past lengthens and the future diminishes, the mind springs an ineluctable slow leak in memory. More often it is like a blowout here and there, in the course of which, we discover that memory, this faculty for remembering and recollecting, is not exactly steel-belted. Forgetfulness becomes a factor in our resourcefulness early in life as well as later. In schoolboy years feats of memory are required for learning biological phylae and important dates, but certain things seem never to fall into a logical scheme: how to spell kwashiorkor, whether my patient's named Tommy have an 'ie' or a 'y' on the end of their names, the definition of autosomal recessive, or the intricacies of Kreb's cycle. And then outside the world of medicine, is it good fences or the absence of them that make good neighbors. These are confusions, not likely to shackle your work or to become serious problems.

Consider the endless irritation of finding information that should be at your fingertips, accessible on demand, just out of reach. Illogical slippage and puncture holes in memory inevitably accelerate as life becomes more crowded with small responsibilities and the manifold details that go along with them. Such pain usually leads to list making, not lists with dramatic entries like, "Lead raid on Tehran, rescue hostages," or "meet with foreign ministers," but more likely to contain entries such as, "pick up laundry," "cash check," or "buy stamps."

I have known one or two people who seem to have what is known in computer science as "random access memory"; their minds are not only well-stocked, but their retrieval systems are nearly perfect. Neighboring quotations, an obscure historical fact, a remote private experience — they need only wish for it and it is there, like the most faithful and efficient watchdog, never sick, and on duty at all times. Others of us feel rather like the man in the old joke who tells a psychiatrist that he has the terrible problem of not being able to remember anything. "When did this problem first arise?" the psychiatrist asks. To which the man replies, "what problem?"

Yet, when it comes to memory, "what problem?" turns out to be a question that invites a look at the state of the art. Nearly every philosopher has adhered to one or more of the many theories of memory. In quite the same way it is one of the great subjects of psychology, fueling many of the experiments devoted to investigating memory. Not only do the theories often conflict, but the experiments seem to have more to do with describing the malfunctions, skewings and tricks of memory than with memory itself. Until recently, as we shall see, scant information has been fielded about the principles of the operation of the memory. New bits and pieces flesh out the concept and new phrases enter into any scientific discussion of memory, but the question of how a particular bit of information is written in the memory remains, essentially a theoretical consideration. I easily forget the anatomical relationship of the inguinal hernia, but quite readily anticipate what happens next in "Gunga Din." Following a story line, seeing a logical progression, or experiencing the impact of drama imprints our memories in a fashion likely to be indelible.

The daily rambling of our consciousness has been estimated to spend 40 percent of its time in the past, 40 percent in the future, and the remainder in the present. As we grow older, the portion of time given to thinking about the past most likely lengthens, even as the past itself lengthens, and that portion given to the future diminishes even as the future itself diminishes.

A distinction, however, must be made between the memory of one's own past and the memory for objects, events and ideas outside oneself. Serious scholarship, such as medicine, depends on a masterful memory of the latter kind along, of course, with keen intelligence. Even this is valueless unless made good by industry, devotion, toil, care, and time to think. This is borne out elsewhere. The Talmud schules of Eastern Europe trained young boys in the daily memorizing and explication of a folio of the Talmud, and an old rabbinic doctrine holds that knowledge of a text is only assured by rereading it 101 times. President Charles Eliot of Harvard admitted that his "gift" for remembering every face and name came from repeating half a dozen times in his mind the name of each new person he met, while looking that person in the face. Many famous feats of memory, in short, have hard work behind them.

The powers of memory are, in spite of recent progress, still mysterious. Most of us wish to pack in too much and the suitcase of memory, filled with all that has gone before, as well as all that is happening now, strains at the straps, unless the feat of memorization can be enhanced. For most of us the condition will be that of a paradox; one condition of remembering is that we should forget.

William James stated it well, "In the practical use of our intellect, forgetting is as important a function as recollecting."

There are limits to the good to be extracted from the best of memories. Dwelling on our finest memories cannot sooth a backache or change a foul mood induced by an argument. But, what an unfathomable sadness not to have fine memories to dwell upon, or to seek the oddments stored therein. Santayana thought, "Inheritance and memory make human stability," and in the *Life of Reason* he wrote: "In endowing us with memory nature has revealed to us a truth utterly unimaginable to the unreflective creation, the truth of mortality." Truly, memory is a process, a process that sparks wonderment at its physiologic and psychologic interrelationships as one of the least known of medicine's frontiers is mastered.

Memory is the psychological function of an organ, the brain. The brain, and the process by which we have access to it, links behavioral science and neurobiology at the molecular level. According to Dr. David A. Drachman of the University of Massachusetts School of Medicine, there must be simultaneous events at three levels each time we incorporate a piece of information into our permanent memory. First, at the neuron level, a switch is thrown that starts a pattern. Next, the pattern spreads to involve the entire brain and finally, the pattern becomes fixed or engrained. The process takes place at an anatomic site with biochemical, physical and physiological interaction.

Information collected in childhood, through the years of schooling and into adulthood becomes an integral part of the brain. Some experiences come in bits or chunks. These have been termed episodic to differentiate them from other experiences that have become known as semantic. Semantic knowledge includes language, rules for behavior or how to swing a golf club; in other words, programs for functioning.

Study of the anatomic basis of memory reveals the vast, perhaps limitless capacity of the brain. The number of dendritic connections of each cell body is a critical aspect of memory. Alterations in the degree of connectivity, such as fewer synapses, is associated with a poorer memory. The brain, on an average, contains 14-20 billion cortical neurons and each of these has about

21

50,000 connections. Each cubic centimeter of brain tissue, no matter the source, contains approximately a trillion connections.

There are a number of questions about these synaptic connections. Can they increase in size? Can new synapses be stimulated? Are there selective increases and decreases in the function of the synapses? If experimental evidence in monkeys is applicable to people, there is great value in rearing children in environments that are intellectually enriching. Monkeys maintained in enriched circumstances have a greater number of large neurons and their cerebral cortices are thicker. Their dendrites are larger, have more crossings and greater branching.

Autopsy studies of older persons killed accidently show more branching of cortical neurons than are found in the young. Yet, the young seem to have more cerebral horsepower. Perhaps the difference is between intelligence in the young and wisdom in the older person. Studies also show selective decreases in some areas of dendritic branching, thought to reflect selective forgetting.

We do not select every sound or every sight for retention in our permanent memory. Some sensory experiences are retained for short-term memory and then allowed to decay. A telephone number, for example, can be retained long enough to dial it; the mechanism has again been deduced from experimental data. According to Dr. Drachman, it has to do with the number of open calcium channels that are located in presynaptic serotonergic neurons. Thus, from an experimental viewpoint, there is an electrolytically related biochemical mechanism that allows a pattern of short-term memory to develop. Long-term memory, on the other hand, seems to be more closely related to flows of sodium, potassium and ATPase as well as to protein metabolism.

Direct memory is enhanced by awareness, attention, reception and perception, and demands structural integrity of the brain. A lesion of the hippocampal area disturbs storage. Sever the corpus callosum and the retrieval process is disrupted. We recognize a Beethoven symphony or a Van Gogh painting by the particular sequence of activation of neurons and synapses; much like the sequence of a movie. If the neurons are activated in an incorrect sequence there is no recognition.

A failure to recognize a familiar song or painting would be alarming, but this is not likely to occur as commonly as the irritations of daily forgetting. This irritation is particularly keen when the forgotten item is a test question, an important person's name, or a crucial meeting. The repercussions can be mildly irritating or seriously compromising, causing one to curse the day he was born with such an inferior piece of equipment. In *Don Quixote* the Man of La Mancha lamented, "My memory is so bad that many times I forget my own name." Few of us are compromised to such a degree. Yet, it's not this end of the spectrum we seek; it's the other, where our memories are trained to a point likely to arouse the envy of colleagues as they listen to a flawless presentation of the differential diagnosis of hypercalcemia.

Books that seek to enhance the memory are usually written by persons who have developed a system to perfection. On the other hand, there are researchers who study the phenomenon and report their findings to others involved in memory research. Some of the limitations of each of these are obvious. Research-oriented books are written in technical language and rarely ever hint toward improvement in memory. Unquestionably, the second type can be successful. Jerry Lucas, a former professional basketball star, has honed the skill to the point of memorization of the Bible using picture-word association. Yet, the limitations of these systems are the length of time they take to be mastered and the restrictions to wide usage in everyday life.

There is a middle ground, one that recognizes principles learned in the laboratory and presents them in non-technical language. Thus, the need is for a general understanding of memory alongside techniques that, once applied, will lead to immediate improvement in memory skills without unrealistic exaggeration or expectations.

Memory research has unearthed three different categories of memory; immediate, short-term and long-term. These systems retain and lose memory, not only in different ways, but also for different spans of time. Consequently, each is used for different purposes and each has methods of enhancement that yield a more bountiful harvest of information.

Immediate Memory

Immediate memory is the remembrance of bits of information just long enought to evaluate whether a response is needed. This facility comes into repeated daily use in the practice of medicine. Consider the number of times sheets of sequential laboratory results are scanned each day. Little thought is given to a blood glucose of 80mg%, but a calcium of 11.5mg% is a different matter. This result demands a close look at chloride, phosphate, total proteins, albumin, globulin and hemoglobin. If these other laboratory values are normal the next step in investigation of the hypercalcemia is planned. Many bits of information were read, considered and forgotten; one demanded a response.

Recording patient histories is a process of sifting and sorting through a pile of mundane information searching for the clue that demands a response. How many times is such a history as this recounted, "It was Tuesday night, no, wait a minute. Was it Wednesday? I'd just finished making a bacon, lettuce and tomato sandwich when Rich Little brought on this guy with a sword swallowing act on *You Asked For It*. I got this burning pain, right here, see, right here. I tell you my nerves are bad. I think that's what it is. I had to lay down and, well, it got a lot worse. I could hear my heart beat in my ear and the pain just kept on going, down to the bottom of my feet and then, all of a sudden, back up to my head. I don't know what it was, but it was a funny feeling. My heart beat funny too, too fast maybe. When I drank something it would start all over again. I'd drink, drink, drink, my stomach was like it didn't have a bottom. My tongue swole up, at first it was black and white. It smarted on the tip end, but now its just white. Feel like I'm smothering when I breath and this grunting sound just came out . . ." The process is one of selection, short retention, response, and decay. Immediate memory is unquestionably a limited system; a response can be made to only one thing at a time; the decay rate is unbelievably swift (one to two seconds); and, furthermore, we are limited to the retention of not more than four items in this system. It is well that memory is not limited to this system.

Competition for attention by two sources of stimulation at the same time is an everyday occurance. You cannot catch the subtleties of a new concept at Grand Rounds while your neighbor in the next seat is telling you about a great movie that's just come to town. One source will be favored and the other will decay within a matter of seconds. Under the same limitations, you cannot switch attention from one novel to another and maintain two separate trains of thought. Awareness is the key to a more effective immediate memory.

Awareness determines what gets plucked from immediate memory before it decays and is lost forever. Awareness also gauges what to discard after a perceived response has been made and what to keep for a longer interval. Awareness will get further attention after we consider what happens with information that is retained in our short-term and long-term memories.

Short-term Memory

Short-term memory is our working memory for those items of information that have been selected for response within the next few seconds or minutes. More items for longer periods can be retained with this system than with immediate memory, but there are limitations with this system as well. Each day it is not unusual to look up different telephone numbers several times and wish to retain the sequence of digits long enough to dial correctly. Rehearsing the numbers over and over insures retention, unless there is interference from another source. Suppose someone calls out random numbers while you are trying to remember a phone number. A digit here or there will inevitably slip. Yet, you will still be able to recall your own phone number because it is in your long-term memory. This emphasizes the distinction between the two systems.

Short-term memory is limited in the number of items that can be retained even through rehearsal. Seven items (plus or minus two) is the upper limit of normal, but practice with eight or nine items succeeds in occasional success or more commonly in wiping out all the items as the system becomes overloaded. The seven item limitation is more easily modified through techniques that will be described in detail later. For the present the basic process will be described.

The process, known as clustering or chunking, is the grouping of similar items into clusters, thereby increasing the total number of items. Your cue to their recall is the cluster, not each individual item. You may, for example, want to remember the following twelve items and, to overcome the limitations of your short-term memory, will have to cluster them: innominate, left carotid and left subclavian arteries, scalenus anterior, scalenus medius, subclavian artery, subclavian vein, brachial plexus and clavicle; ophthalmic, mandibular and maxillary nerves. The cluster; branches of the arch of the aorta, structures that cross the first rib, and branches of the trigeminal nerve. These clusters are well within the capability of short-term memory and at the moment of recall of each cluster the items under that category will spring to mind. So much for short-term memory for the moment. Methods of enhancement will be considered as we move along, but let's turn to the characteristics, limitations and potential of long-term memory.

Long-term Memory

Long-term memory is memory for information that was acquired minutes to years in the past. Such information has obviously not been rehearsed during all this time and yet it can be recalled. The ease and success of that recall depends upon the manner of organization of that bit of information. The capacity to store information is limitless, but the clue to improving the effectiveness of long-term memory lies in the way the facts we wish to retain are organized. The vastness of the storage capacity encourages retention of more and more information and it is true, as with most functions, the more we use long-term memory the greater our skill at organizing and integrating the information. A well-organized long-term memory not only facilitates retrieval, but it eases the pain of learning and memorizing new material.

In an earlier time consciousness or awareness was stimulated constantly, except when asleep. It was a matter of survival. But those things seen, heard, felt, smelled or thought were discarded unless they were a threat to survival. Society has evolved into communities that insure a reasonable degree of safety through law enforcement, leaving our senses free to experience and select out information of great variety. Much of what we experience is discarded, but our attention is focused by our interests and we select a bit here and a piece there to be savored in short-term memory or passed directly into long-term memory.

While savoring that morsel in short-term memory, perhaps a special point made during a lecture, the rest of the lecture is sliding by until the decision is made to drop the information or retain it in long-term memory. Of course, the process proceeds automatically and the ability to recall that bit of information depends on the skill with which it was organized into what is already known. Sometimes we mentally reorganize things to introduce order from chaos, thereby facilitating the process of recall. It is our purpose to disencumber the process in the remaining chapters.

Chapter 3

Mnemonics:

Blood and Blood Chemistry

First, do no harm.

> — Oath of the Hindu Physician

No physician is really good before he has killed one or two patients.

> — Old Hindu Proverb

The art of medicine consists of introducing a body of which we know little into another, of which we know still less.

> — A Paraphrasing of Voltaire
> as used by Dr. Alfred Stille.

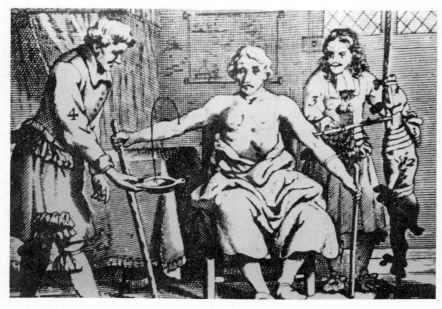

An etching demonstrating a transfusion from lamb to man and the act of blood-letting which was thought to be a necessary procedure to make room for the incoming blood.

Causes of Elevated Platelet Counts

Elevated platelet counts can be subdivided into two groups. When the count is between 400,000 and 800,000 per mm.^{3} and the elevation is transient, the term thrombocytosis is used. Thrombocythemia refers to a sustained elevation above 800,000 per mm.^{3} Such high counts are noted predominantly in myeloproliferative disorders and are associated with an enlarged spleen. Counts exceeding one million per mm.^{3} may lead to thrombotic episodes. Hemorrhage may also occur and correlates with platelet size, being most common in conditions which have large, bizarre platelet forms and megakaryocyte fragments. Clotted blood collected from patients with high platelet counts may display spurious hyperkalemia resulting from normal release of potassium from the increased platelet mass.

Acrostic for Elevated Platelet Counts:
H-I   P-L-A-T-E-L-E-T-S*

Hemorrhage (acute) — The mechanism of thrombocytosis here appears to be overproduction rather than lengthening of survival time. In response to acute hemorrhage, however, there may be the additional release of platelets from the spleen or the lungs.

Inflammatory disorders — (such as rheumatoid arthritis, rheumatic fever, inflammatory bowel disease, sarcoid, osteomyelitis) cause increased production of platelets, possibly mediated by a platelet stimulating factor.

Polycythemia vera — The bleeding tendency seen in polycythemia vera is due to both abnormal platelet aggregation and a distended vasculature secondary to increased blood volume.

Leukemia — In acute leukemia the platelet count is usually moderately or greatly decreased. However, in the myeloproliferative syndrome, chronic granulocytic leukemia, half the patients will have platelet counts above 450,000 per mm.^{3}

Anemia (iron deficiency) — Thrombocytosis occurring with iron deficiency anemia is corrected by iron therapy. Hemolytic anemia is also associated with elevated platelet counts.

Tumor — Elevated platelet counts are commonly seen with many carcinomas and occasionally precede the diagnosis of malignancy.

Essential thrombocythemia — a myeloproliferative disorder, is characterized by normal erythrocyte and leukocyte counts, and very high platelet counts. Bleeding and thrombotic complications are frequent.

Lymphoma — Hodgkin's disease and other lymphomas, like carcinoma, can be associated with high platelet counts.

Epinephrine and Exercise — like acute hemorrhage, cause release of platelets from storage areas. Postoperative thrombocytosis, other than post splenectomy cases, is probably caused by this mechanism.

Toxin or recovery from Toxic State (Vincristine, alcohol withdrawal).

Splenectomy — results in thrombocytosis which commences within two weeks of surgery and lasts approximately three months.

Splenomegaly

The spleen, with its labyrinthine microstructure, functions partly as a clearing house, exposing the blood elements to immunologic, metabolic and physical obstacles. It culls out defective red cells, removes unsightly Heinz bodies and malarial parasites, and garners platelets as they careen down the malpighian corpuscles. In this way it serves the body as an in vivo plasmapheresis lab.

An Acrostic for the Causes of Splenomegaly:
P-L-A-S-M-A-P-H-A-R-E-S-I-S   L-A-B*
(please excuse the spelling)

Portal hypertension — no matter the cause, can produce congestive splenomegaly (Banti's syndrome) which is associated with the signs of hypersplenism and gastrointestinal bleeding.

Lupus (SLE) — Ten to twenty percent of patients with lupus have enlarged spleens. As with the other causes listed here, it may be associated with pancytopenia and a hyperactive bone marrow (hypersplenism). (See mnemonic for SLE criteria p. 133)

Amyloid — may lead to splenomegaly, though isolated hepatic enlargement is found more frequently.

Sarcoid — can present with features mimicking a lymphorecticular disorder with generalized lymphadenopathy. Twenty five percent of affected patients have splenomegaly.

Mycobacteria (and Malaria) — Large spleens are more common in malaria than in tuberculosis. Splenic rupture is a rare but catastrophic complication of malaria.

Abscess (splenic abscess) — Tender splenomegaly with peritoneal irritation occurs in lower pole abscesses of the spleen, whereas upper pole abscesses lead to pleuritic pain with left pleural effusion and diaphragmatic elevation. Abscesses develop as a result of bacteremia, previous splenic infarction, perforation of a neighboring visceral organ, or extension of abdominal carcinoma.

Polycythemia vera (and related myeloproliferative syndromes) — Present in seventy five percent of patients with polycythemia vera and virtually all cases of agnogenic myeloid metaplasia, splenomegaly is the most useful physical finding in distinguishing primary from secondary polycythemia.

Histoplasmosis — Disseminated disease, which occurs most often in infants and the elderly, involves multiple organs including adrenals, brain, kidney, lung, lymph nodes, liver, skin and spleen.

Anemia (hemolytic) — In certain varieties of hemolytic anemia, such as hereditary spherocytosis and autoimmune hemolytic anemias, the spleen's efficiency as a filter becomes a detriment to the body. In these cases, splenectomy may dramatically improve the anemic state.

Rheumatoid arthritis — Ten percent of patients with rheumatoid arthritis have splenomegaly. Some will display widespread lymphadenopathy, mimicking lymphoma. Felty's syndrome, the triad of rheumatoid arthritis, splenomegaly and neutropenia usually occurs in patients with long-standing disease.

Endocarditis — Subacute bacterial endocarditis commonly causes splenomegaly when splenic infarction complicates the course of the disease. Left upper quadrant abdominal pain and a friction rub are the hallmarks of this complication.

Syphilis — Late benign syphilis may produce splenomegaly usually in association with gummatous hepatitis.

Infectious mono — Fifty percent of patients with mononucleosis will manifest splenomegaly. It is most prominent during the second and third week of illness.

Shistosomiasis — Splenomegaly can occur during the acute serum-sickness-like illness (Katayama syndrome) or result from the late-stage fibrosis of the portal system with concomitant portal hypertension.

Leukemias and **L**ymphomas — This group, along with the myeloproliferative syndromes, composes the major etiologies for truly massive splenomegaly.

Aneurysm of the splenic artery — Occurring most often in elderly women, splenic artery aneurysm may cause cramping abdominal pain or be completely asymptomatic. On physical exam a pulsatile enlarged spleen and left upper quadrant bruit may be present.

Brucella — A tender, enlarged spleen is seen most often in severe cases of acute disease. In chronic disease x-ray may reveal calcified granulomata in the liver and spleen.

This list fails to include a few disorders which cause splenomegaly (cytomegalovirus, kala-azar, lipoidoses). The following mnemonic is more general and thus, all-inclusive.

Mechanisms of Splenic Enlargement:
Acrostic — S-P-L-E-E-N

Sequestration — (e.g. hereditary spherocytosis).

Proliferation — (e.g. mononucleosis, malaria).

Lipid — (e.g. Niemann-Pick, Gaucher's).

Engorgement — (e.g. portal hypertension, trauma).

<u>E</u>ndowment (e.g. congenital hemangiomas).

i<u>N</u>vasion — (e.g. lymphoma, granulomatous disorders).

> The causes of all diseases are to be found in the blood."
> — Hebrew Proverb

Lymphocytosis

Lymphocytosis is defined as greater than 4,500 lymphocytes per mm.[3] The word "lymph" originates from the Greek word for marriageable girl and is directly related to the word "nymph." Nymphs were minor deities of rivers, lakes, forests and moist fertile areas. The adjective "lymphatic" was used by ancient Greek physicians as a synonym for "phlegmatic," a term attributable to those with moist and torpid temperaments, uninterested in gastric or venereal delights.

Acronym for the Causes of Lymphocytosis:
P-H-L-E-G-M-A-T-I-C   M-I-S-S*

<u>P</u>ertussis — Although the characteristic whoop is usually absent in children less than six months old, its presence along with paroxysms of coughing strongly suggest the diagnosis. Increased leukocyte counts (occasionally over 100,000) are composed primarily of mature lymphocytes. Rarely are circulating atypical lymphocytes seen.

<u>H</u>epatitis (infectious) — Atypical lymphocytes (usually less than twelve percent of the white cell count) are common in the acute phase of hepatitis A and B. The lymphocytosis may be preceded by transient neutropenia and lymphopenia.

<u>L</u>eukemia — Acute lymphocytic leukemia usually produces lymphocytosis accompanied by granulocytopenia, thrombocytopenia and anemia. In chronic lymphocytic leukemia there is an increase in circulating immature lymphocytes (most often between 10,000 and 150,000 per mm.[3]). The leukemic phase of mycosis fungoides, a T-cell lymphoma, also displays a lymphocytosis.

<u>E</u>nterovirus — infections causing epidemics of diarrheal illness have been associated with lymphocytosis, especially in chil-

dren.

German measles (rubella) — in its prodromal stage closely resembles infectious mononucleosis. The rash in rubella, however, invariably affects the face. This distinguishes it from mono, in which the skin is involved over the trunk but not over the face.

Mumps — causes painful, nonerythematous, euthermic parotid swelling associated with a relative lymphocytosis. The total white blood cell count is usually normal. This is in sharp contrast to bacterial parotitis which is warm, red and accompanied by a leukocytosis with a leftward shift.

Adrenal insufficiency — In uncomplicated Addison's disease, anemia is mild and may be masked by hemoconcentration. The leukocyte count is often low normal with a relative lymphocytosis.

Thyrotoxicosis — Lymphocytosis is frequently present in the thyrotoxic individual. Occasionally, the cervical lymph nodes will be enlarged and the spleen tip will be palpable.

Infectious mononucleosis — Predominant features during the active phase of disease are lymphadenopathy, fever and pharyngitis (90-95 percent of patients), splenomegaly (more than 50 percent), and hepatomegaly (approximately 50 percent). Atypical lymphocyte counts peak at one week's time, constituting greater than twenty percent of the leukocyte count.

Cytomegalovirus — a herpes virus, can cause an illness easily confused with infectious mono. Common features of the two infections include splenomegaly, atypical lymphocytes and hepatomegaly. (Distinguishing it from mono, CMV mononucleosis is not usually accompanied by cervical lymphadenopathy or pharyngitis).

Mycobacteria (tuberculosis) — In disseminated tuberculosis the white cell count may be low, normal or high. Leukocytosis is most common in tuberculous pneumonia, meningitis, and miliary tuberculosis. In miliary disease, a leukemoid reaction may be noted.

Infectious lymphocytosis — a benign disorder of children, is usually associated with the symptoms of an upper respiratory tract infection. The leukocytosis seen in the disease consists mainly of small mature lymphocytes. Adenopathy is minimal, splenomegaly is not present and the heterophile antibody test is negative.

Splenectomy — Both thrombocytosis and lymphocytosis are sequelae of splenectomy.

Serum sickness and similar allergic or autoimmune reactions cause neutropenia and lymphopenia in the acute phase. During recovery a conspicuous lymphocytosis may occur. Convalescence from a variety of illnesses may be associated with a high lymphocyte count. Prior to the advent of antibiotics, lymphocytosis was used as a clinical index of recovery from infectious diseases.

Notable exclusions from this list are brucellosis and syphilis.

Eosinophilia

In normal subjects the total eosinophil count remains below 450 cells per mm^3 and is usually in the range of 100 to 150 cells per mm^3. The word eosinophil is derived from ''EOS'', the Greek name for the goddess of the rosy-colored dawn. Her Roman name was Aurora.

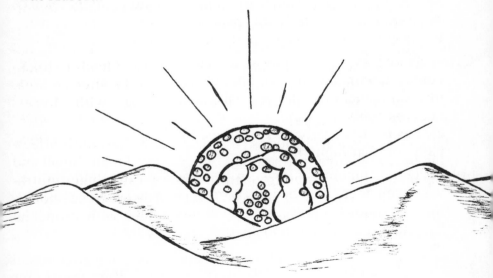

Art: C. Pedley
Concept: R. Bloomfield

A Mnemonic for the Causes of Eosinophilia:
A-S P-U-R-E A-S L-I-G-H-T*

<u>A</u>llergic disorders — are the commonest causes for eosinophilia. Eosinophilia in these cases is usually mild, although in symptomatic asthma it is consistently elevated. Some other examples include seasonal rhinitis, hypersensitivity pneumonitis and serum sickness. Some further examples overlap the second group of diseases listed here;

<u>S</u>kin disorders — including atopic eczematous dermatitis, Stevens-Johnson syndrome, psoriasis, dermatitis herpetiformis and pemphigus vulgaris.

<u>P</u>arasites — The extent of eosinophilia in parasitic infestation is related to the activity and the invasiveness of the infection. The most frequent causative organisms are the helminths, including strongyloides, ascarias, toxocariasis (visceral larva migrans), hookworms, trichinosis and filariasis.

<u>U</u>lcerative colitis and

<u>R</u>egional enteritis — may cause mild eosinophilia. A rarer gastrointestinal disorder more closely associated with eosinophilia, however, is eosinophilic gastroenteritis. This disease affects the stomach and small bowel, is accompanied by a marked peripheral eosinophilia, and may cause steatorrhea and protein losing enteropathy.

<u>E</u>osinophilic fasciitis — is an entity which characteristically occurs hours to days after physical exertion and leads to thickening and immobility of the skin overlying the affected area. Eosinophilia is usually present along with hypergammaglobulinemia.

<u>A</u>rteritis — Polyarteritis nodosa is a necrotizing vasculitis affecting multiple organs in young to middle aged men. Small and middle-sized arteries frequently show eosinophilic infiltration on histologic examination. A related disorder, eosinophilic granulomatous vasculitis, is associated with bronchial asthma and an allergic history.

<u>S</u>arcoid — A disease characterized by non-caseating granulomas, can affect multiple organs throughout the body (most com-

37

monly lung, lymph nodes, skin, eyes, liver and spleen). Frequently anemia, leukopenia, eosinophilia and an elevated sedimentation rate are found.

Loeffler's syndrome (and associated PIE syndromes) — Secondary eosinophilic reactions of the lung may be provoked by toxins, allergy, autoimmune disease, granulomatous disorders or malignancy. Pulmonary infiltrates and eosinophilia (PIE) including Loeffler's transient migratory pulmonic infiltrates, are terms reserved for primary idiopathic eosinophilic reactions of the lung.

Inherited — Though occasionally seen as a familial anomaly, eosinophilia should prompt a search for more common causes.

Goodpasture's — This necrotizing glomerulitis demonstrates circulating glomerular basement membrane antibodies that lead to a linear immuno-fluorescent pattern on renal biopsy. Also characteristic is life threatening pulmonary hemorrhage. Polyarteritis nodosa may also present with renal failure, pulmonary hemorrhage and eosinophilia, but GBM antibodies are not found.

Hypereosinophilic syndrome — has alternatively been called Loeffler's fibroplastic endocarditis and eosinophilic leukemia. The criteria for diagnosis include an eosinophil count greater than 1500 per mm^3, no evidence of other causes of eosinophilic disease states, and signs of organ involvement (most commonly cardiac or central nervous system).

Tumor — Malignancies which are associated with eosinophilia include solid tumors, especially those of mucin-secreting origin, lymphomas, myeloproliferative disorders, acute lymphocytic leukemia and immunoblastic lymphadenopathy (a special subset of lymphomas).

Three Four

The numbers 3 and 4 serve as a mnemonic key to several relationships in hematology.

1.**34** cc^3 of oxygen is carried by each gram of hemoglobin.

3.4 is the average number of nuclear lobes per neutrophil after counting 100 cells (if in the process of counting one should see more than three neutrophils with five lobes or a single cell with six lobes, the presumptive diagnosis of megaloblastic anemia can be made).

3.4 milligrams of iron is contained in each gram of hemoglobin.

34 milligrams of bilirubin are produced from each gram of hemoglobulin.

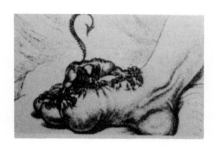

The gout

Hyperuricemia

Major complications of hyperuricemia include gout and nephrolithiasis both of which may occur in the absence of elevated uric acid levels. Whether presented with these striking consequences of hyperuricemia which demand definitive therapy or with asymptomatic hyperuricemia, in which the need for treatment remains controversial, the clinician must consider the possible causes and exacerbating factors.

Abecedarius: The ABC's of Hyperuricemia (causes and associated states)*

A — **A**cidosis inhibits renal secretion of urates.

B — **B**lood cells lysis — hemolytic anemia chronically produces a secondary rise in nucleic acid turnover.

C — **C**ancer — increased nucleic acid turnover also occurs in myeloproliferative disorders, lymphomas, multiple myeloma, and cancer therapy (both chemotherapy and radiation therapy).

D — **D**rugs (and toxins) — Alcohol in excess results in accumulation of lactate which, in turn, inhibits renal secretion of urates. Salicylates in low doses and pyrazinamide also decrease tubular secretion. Diuretics, on the other hand, increase tubular reabsorption. Lead, by producing chronic hemolysis, also causes elevated serum urate.

E — **E**nzymatic defects — The commonest enzyme defect causing hyperuricemia is glucose-6-phosphatase deficiency in Von Gierke's disease. Other rarer causes include Lesch-Nyhan syndrome, increased glutathione reductase activity and, (take a breath now), glutamine phosphoribosylpyrophosphate deficiency.

F — **F**at and **F**amine — Obesity, the hyerlipidemias (types III, IV and V) and starvation are associated with high uric acid levels.

G — **G**ranulomatous disease — In sarcoid, the serum uric acid level may be elevated even in the absence of renal disease.

H — **H**ypothyroidism and **H**ypoadrenalism produce decreased renal perfusion and subsequent hyperuricemia.

I — **I**diopathic — Primary idiopathic hyperuricemia is a complex category made up of patients, one third of whom overproduce uric acid, another third who underexcrete urate, and a remaining third who demonstrate a combination of both factors.

J — **J**ava — Coffee, tea and cocoa contain methylxanthines that may be converted into uric acid, although clear evidence for this phenomenon is lacking.

K — **K**idney failure — Decreased renal perfusion or renal mass lead to hyperuricemia.

This list lacks two other causes; psoriasis and purine-rich diet (rarely causative).

Hyponatremia

The origin of the word "natrium" is controversial. Some sources are convinced it comes from an ancient lake called Natrion in which the sodium concentration was so high that crystals formed at the shoreline.

A primary goal in examination of the hyponatremic patient is deducing the relative amount of extracellular fluid present. Edema usually belies excess total body sodium; whereas decreased skin turgor, tachycardia and orthostatic hypotension reveal decreased total body sodium.

Mnemonic: For Causes of Hyponatremia
   P-I-S-S: (dilutional hyponatremia)
     S-I-A-D-H: (low total body sodium)
       H-H-H: (increased body water and sodium)*

Psychogenic water intoxication

Iatrogenic water administration
      and the

Syndrome of inappropriate ADH are causes
      for

Sodium content which is normal in a body with too much water (dilutional).

Salt losing nephropathy,

Intestinal loss of fluid,

Addison's disease,
      and

Diuretic therapy
      cause

Hyponatremia associated with a deficit of body sodium.

Heart failure
      and

Hepatic insufficiency (cirrhosis)
      cause

Hyponatremia associated with both increased body water and
   sodium.

Anion Gap Acidosis

   The difference in mEq per liter between the major extracellular anions (Cl − and HCO_3 −) and the principal extracellular cation (Na +) is termed the anion gap. The anion gap is normally less
than 12-14 mEq per liter. Any acid that contains hydrogen ions
and a dissociated anion can produce a widened anion gap.

   Ion comes from the Greek words meaning "to go". Anions,
the negatively charged ions, pass into a positively charged anode.

Mnemonic for the Causes of Anion Gap Acidosis:
M-A-D-E   A   P-L-U-S*
 −   →   +

Methanol — is an ingredient in sterno, solox, antifreeze, paint
   remover and denatured ethyl alcohol. Symptoms (including
   headache, central nervous system depression, abdominal
   pain and visual disturbance) are delayed in their appearance
   for 12-24 hours, the time required for accumulation of toxic
   metabolites (esp. formaldehyde). Kussmaul's respirations, in
   spite of severe acidosis, are frequently absent.

Aspirin (salicylates) — Symptoms of salicylate poisoning, poorly
   correlated with plasma levels, include vertigo, tinnitus, headache, diarrhea and mental confusion. Toxic levels produce
   hyperventilation and respiratory alkalosis. With progressive
   accumulation of acid metabolites, however, respiratory depression may ensue, compounding the acidosis.

Diabetic ketoacidosis — The nitroprusside reaction detects the
   ketones acetoacetate and acetone by becoming a distinctly
   purple color. However, betahydroxybutyrate, the predominant ketone body, does not react. Its concentration can be
   roughly estimated at three times the concentration of acetoacetate. The sum of the three ketones will roughly equal the
   anion gap in this clinical situation.

Ethylene glycol — found in antifreeze, causes symptomatology
   similar to alcohol intoxication shortly after ingestion. Asso-

ciated signs include hypothermia, bradycardia and tachypnea. Death may occur due to respiratory failure, pulmonary edema, or after the acute stage, as a consequence of hepatic and renal necrosis.

<u>A</u>lcoholic ketoacidosis is usually mild and can be associated with mild elevation of serum glucose (usually less than 330 mg/dl) or with hypoglycemia. Starvation and dehydration are the usual prerequisites to this clinical picture.

<u>P</u>araldehyde — pharmacologically similar to alcohol, is a generally safe hypnotic medication which suppresses alcohol withdrawal symptoms. On exposure to light, however, it decomposes to the toxic acetaldehyde.

<u>L</u>actic acidosis may complicate many disease states such as sepsis and shock, diabetic ketoacidosis and phenformin therapy, hepatic insufficiency and peritoneal dialysis in the presence of liver disease, leukemia and glucose-6-phosphatase deficiency.

<u>U</u>remia — As the glomerular filtration rate falls below fifty percent of normal, the kidney's ability to excrete the body's daily acid load becomes inadequate. Consequently, sulfates and phosphates accumulate and widen the anion gap.

<u>S</u>tarvation — through its production of ketoacids, leads to anion gap acidosis.

Hypokalemia

Hypokalemia may result from gastrointestinal losses of potassium, inadequate dietary intake, renal potassium losses, or intracellular potassium shifts. Gastrointestinal losses are the most common cause of hypokalemia. Among renal etiologies of potassium loss, diuretic use is the most frequent.

Acrostic for Causes of Potassium Depletion and Hypokalemia:

I'-L-L   A-D-D   P-O-T-A-S-S-I-U-M*

<u>I</u>nsulin effect — Insulin lack leads to potassium and sodium depletion through several mechanisms in patients with diabetic

ketoacidosis. Insulin administration serves to transport potassium into cells along with glucose, thus lowering serum potassium without depleting the body of this cation.

Leukemia with Lysozymuria — In mono- and myelomonocytic leukemia, lysozyme (muramidase) may be associated with proteinuria, glomerulotubular dysfunction and renal potassium loss.

Liddle's disease — A renal tubular defect is the reason for potassium wasting in this rare inherited disorder.

Alkalosis — tends to shift potassium intracellularly creating hypokalemia. Acidosis does the opposite, favoring hyperkalemia. In acidosis, however, total body potassium depletion may ensue in spite of normal or high potassium levels due to increased renal excretion.

Diuretics — The potassium sparing diuretics such as triamterene and spironolactone are compounds in this group that do not provoke hypokalemia.

Diarrhea — from any cause will result in potassium depletion. The concomitant loss of bicarbonate produces an acidosis which may mask the deficit by producing cellular shifts of potassium.

Periodic paralysis — Sudden shifts of potassium to the intracellular compartment are responsible for the hypotonia and paralysis seen in this rare familial disorder. Although a high carbohydrate meal or exercise may provoke an attack, usually no precipitating event can be identified.

Oral loss (vomiting) — The potassium concentration of vomitus is low (5-10 mEq liter). The hypokalemia which occurs in this setting can be traced mainly to two factors. First, volume depletion will cause secondary hyperaldosteronism. Additionally, the metabolic alkalosis will result in increased delivery of bicarbonate to the renal tubules. Both of these factors produce renal potassium secretion.

Tubular acidosis (RTA) — RTA is one of the few settings in which a severe acidosis and hypokalemia coexist. Both type I (distal tubule) and type II (proximal tubule) result in potassium depletion. A listing of etiologies is provided in the appendix, p. 212

Adrenocortial excess — as found in ACTH producing tumors, exogenous corticosteroids, Cushing's syndrome and primary aldosteronism cause potassium wastage.

Secondary hyperaldosteronism — as seen in Barter's syndrome, nephrosis, cirrhosis, malignant hypertension and licorice ingestion also cause renal potassium loss.

Starvation (deficient dietary intake of potassium) — It takes 10 to 14 days for renal mechanisms to compensate for inadequate potassium intake. During that time, renal potassium excretion may lead to sizable deficits.

Ileostomy and

Ureterosigmoidostomy — may produce hypokalemia. In the latter condition, colonic absorption of sodium chloride leads to secretion of potassium and bicarbonate. Consequently the patient may display hyperchloremic hypokalemic acidosis.

Milk of Magnesia (laxative abuse) — an overlooked cause of hypokalemia, laxative abuse is a habit that may be adamantly denied by abusing patients.

Hypercalcemia

In order to correctly interpret the serum calcium, it is important to remember several variables which may affect its blood level. About 0.8 mg of calcium is bound to 1.0 gram of serum protein (albumin and globulin). Therefore, the presence of protein abnormalities may alter the measured calcium level without representing true hyper- or hypocalcemia. False elevations occur after prolonged venous stasis prior to blood drawing. Since erythrocytes absorb calcium, levels may be spuriously low when blood has been allowed to stand for long periods without the separation of serum.

The Latin word for calcium was "calx," which meant lime or rubble. The name "calcaneus" for the bone in the heel was arrived at probably because of the bone's resemblance to a slab of limestone.

Acronym for the Symptoms and Signs seen with Hypercalcemia:
U-N-D-E-R   M-U-C-H   C-A-L-X*

<u>U</u>rinary frequency (due to inability to maximally concentrate urine).

<u>N</u>ausea

<u>D</u>ysesthesias

<u>E</u>mesis

<u>R</u>enalithiasis (diffuse nephrocalcinosis may also occur).

<u>M</u>yalgias

<u>U</u>lcers (increased calcium stimulates gastrin secretion leading to peptic ulceration).

<u>C</u>onstipation

<u>H</u>ypertension (may be secondary to renal parenchymal damage or to a vasoconstrictive effect of calcium).

<u>C</u>oma

<u>A</u>rrhythmia (hypercalcemia shortens the refractory period and slows conduction leading, at times, to the development of PVC's, ventricular tachycardia and ventricular fibrillation).

<u>L</u>ethargy

<u>X</u>erostomia (is in part due to dehydration from the associated polyuria).

This list fails to include bone pain.

With regard to the etiologies of hypercalcemia a categorical approach using the immunoglobulin classes as clues, aids in the recall of the major causes.

Causes of Hypercalcemia:
Mnemonic: Immunoglobulins — G-A-M-E-D*

<u>I</u>mmunoglobulins — Immobilization.

G — <u>G</u>ranulomatous diseases — sarcoid, tuberculosis, berylliosis, coccidioidomycosis.

A — <u>A</u>rtifactual — hyperproteinemia, venous stasis during collection.

M — **M**alignancy — solid tumors, multiple myeloma, lymphoma, leukemia.

E — **E**ndocrine causes — primary hyperparathyroidism, secondary hyperparathyroidism, hyperthyroidism.

D - **D**rugs — vitamin-D intoxication, thiazides, milk alkali, vitamin-A intoxication, magnesium excess.

The more complex acrostic which follows delineates specific causes of hypercalcemia.

Acronym for the Causes of Hypercalcemia:
S-U-P-R-A   A-C-T-I-V-E   P-T-H*

Sarcoid — Approximately twenty percent of patients with sarcoid have hypercalcemia associated with increased intestinal absorption of this mineral.

Uremia — Serum calcium levels are usually depressed in patients with chronic renal failure due to hyperphosphatemia. However, secondary hyperparathyroidism may develop after long-standing renal failure resulting in hypercalcemia. Additionally, after dialysis or transplantation, transient hypercalcemia may be noted accompanying rapid decrements of serum phosphate.

Pagets disease — a chronic, usually asymptomatic bone disease, is characterized by increased bone resorption, elevated alkaline phosphatase (correlated with disease activity) and usually focal involvement (especially pelvis, skull, vertebral column and femur). Calcium is usually normal unless immobility complicates the disease.

Renal transplantation — Hypercalcemia may occur days to weeks after transplantation and occasionally persists for years, resulting in bony complications (e.g. aseptic necrosis of the femoral head). The usual underlying problem is secondary hyperparathyroidism.

Addison's disease — The cause for elevated serum calcium in adrenal insufficiency is probably a consequence of hypovolemia.

Alkali (milk-alkali syndrome) — Ingestion of milk and alkali (or

47

carbonate antacids) causes hypercalcemia and renal phosphate retention resulting in hyperphosphatemia and alkalosis.

Carcinoma — Malignancy and primary hyperparathyroidism constitute the commonest causes for hypercalcemia. Breast and lung are the frequent sites of the responsible carcinomas. Although skeletal metastases may be present, a PTH-like substance can be produced by different cancers (especially lung and kidney).

Thiazides — Long term administration of thiazides may cause hypercalcemia by decreasing tubular excretion of the cation or by increasing tubular reabsorption.

Idiopathic infantile hypercalcemia (or alternatively Immobilization) — This unusual pediatric disorder has been attributed to hypersensitivity to the effects of vitamin-D.

Vitamin-D intoxication — 1,25 dehydroxycholecalciferol increases intestinal absorption of calcium and phosphate, facilitates bone mineralization and is required for PTH to act in bone resorption. Daily doses above 100,000 units for many months leads to hypercalcemia. The hypercalcemia is acutely responsive to glucocorticoid medication but persists for weeks to months when withdrawal of vitamin-D is effected without other forms of therapy.

E prostaglandin — produced by some tumors (e.g. hypernephroma) stimulates resorption of bone. A prostaglandin inhibitor, indomethacin, may lower calcium levels in this situation.

Plasmacytoma — Multiple myeloma, an immunoglobulin secreting neoplasm, also has been shown to secrete an osteoclastic activating factor which provokes the characteristic osteolytic lesions of bone.

Thyrotoxicosis — Excess thyroid hormone increases bone turnover and, in this way, is postulated to raise serum calcium. This unusual complication of hyperthyroidism is usually reversed by antithyroid treatment. If calcium remains elevated it is well to remember the association of hyperthyroidism and . . .

Hyperparathyroidism — Primary hyperparathyroidism is characterized by elevations of calcium, mild hyperchloremic acidosis, mildly depressed or normal serum phosphate and elevated PTH levels. Renal and bone disease, two insidious complications are the main indications for parathyroidectomy.

Chapter 4

OBSERVATION

Our Task

To wrest from nature the secrets which have perplexed philosophers in all ages, to track to their sources the causes of disease, to correlate the vast stores of knowledge, that they may be quickly available for the prevention and cure of disease — these are our ambitions. To carefully observe the phenomena of life in all its phases, normal and perverted, to make perfect that most difficult of all the arts, the art of observation, to call to aid the science of experimentation, to cultivate the reasoning faculty, so as to be able to know the true from the false — these are our methods. To prevent disease, to relieve suffering and to heal the sick — this is our work. The profession in truth is a sort of guild or brotherhood, any member of which can take up his calling in any part of the world and find brethren whose language and methods and whose aims are identical with his own.

Osler
Chauvinism in Medicine, 1902.

Each one of us, however old, is still an undergraduate in the school of experience. When a man thinks he has graduated he becomes a public menace.

John Chalmers Da Costa

The physician's level of knowledge is never satisfactory. Information from the medical world accumulates at too great a rate to be assimilated. The infinite variation of people confounds a naive clinician. The dissimilarity of red blood cells, estimated to be 10 to the twentieth power, emphasizes this variety. Disease processes can be catagorized, but when housed in different bodies that defy catagorization, the diversity spoils any sense of uniformity in the way diseases present. The physician who would be an effective clinician must seek ways to hone his skill of awareness to a keen edge.

The level of diagnostic astuteness should be at its highest ever. The appeal of the laboratory as a diagnostic instrument, however, overshadows the wisdom of a basic grounding in the effectiveness of extracting the story of a sickness from the patient and finding the evidence on his body with the use of eye, ear and hand.

This approach has stood the test of time from the days of Hippocrates to the present. One might suppose that medicine steadily groped its way towards enlightment and effectiveness. It is true that the progress of medicine has had such cries of success, but many of the discoveries in biology and medicine have been come upon unexpectedly, or at least had an element of chance in them, especially the most important and revolutionary ones. Although we cannot deliberately evoke that will-o-the-wisp, chance, we can be on the alert for it, prepare ourselves to recognize it and profit from it when it comes. Clinical medicine and basic research are well served by the training of powers of observation and cultivation of attitudes that stimulate us to constantly be on the alert for the unexpected and to habitually examine every clue that chance presents. Discoveries are made by giving attention to the slightest clue.

Most of us practice medicine under the direction of principles and assumptions which had their origins in the comparatively recent past and it is almost impossible to trace back a direct line of thought much beyond the seventeenth century. From that date on, the descriptions of the body and its processes are at least comparable with our own. The insights of the scientific renaissance did not have important practical consequences until the beginning of this century. It is possible, however, to recognize the reasoning involved in those astute founding observations.

Even so, medicine's contribution to human welfare, outside of methods of improved sewage control and cleaner food and water, were not greatly significant until the middle of the twentieth century. Heroic procedures and the discovery of new drugs, though often given credit for a great leap forward, do not benefit the majority of the people. Medicine has gained a distinguishing mark in the past twenty-five years; it is not that its practitioners are armed with an arsenal of antibiotics and new cardiac drugs, but that they are furnished with a comprehensive and unprecedented understanding of how the body works, how it survives and protects itself. Before we are able to direct these physiologic processes, however, we must be certain to have gained an adequate understanding of the patient and his relationship to the physician.

The Physician's Role

"Physicians, get neither name nor fame by the pricking of wheals or the picking out thistles, or by laying of plaisters to the scratch of a pin; every old woman can do this. But if they would have a name and a fame, if they will have it quickly, they must do some great and desperate cures. Let them fetch one to life that was dead, let them recover one to his wits that was mad, let them make one that was born blind to see, or let them give ripe wits to a fool — these are notable cures, and he that can do thus, if he doth thus first, he shall have the name and fame he deserves; he may lie abed till noon."

John Bunyan

Physician's skills are devoted to two duties, namely, to preserve the quality of life and to prevent or ameliorate suffering. In clinical practice these two duties are carried out in a relationship between one patient and one doctor. Although medical practice is a transaction between two individuals, each is individual only in a corporate sense. The physician's efforts are complemented and enhanced by contributions made by various medical specialists including nurses, technicians, social workers, and pharmacists. Similarly, the patient may have a spouse, children, neighbors, employers, and others attached to him in various degrees. These persons are involved in the patient's disease, some centrally, others peripherally, and the waves of their concern reverberate, in some cases with far more aggravation than the patient's own illness.

In such a setting the physician begins his search of the

patient's life for clues from the past and present in his desire to modify the patient's future. Not only is the patient helped, the physician's knowledge of the disease in question is broadened, his curiosity is aroused and his mind stimulated by the puzzle to be unraveled. His understanding of human nature deepens with each case.

Early in their careers physicians learn medicine by watching and participating in the transactions between a patient and an experienced clinician. In this setting learning is not always conscious and the cerebral processes by which physicians make diagnoses or exercise subtle clinical judgements are not clearly definable. It is clear, however, that at such times the physicians are responding to sensory cues of which they are unaware. They are reasoning on the basis of items of information perceived unconsciously. This type of cerebration is called "intuition." Studies of intuition show that it is based on unrecognized and sometimes fragmentary memory. Albert Einstein said of his own creative processes, "The really valuable thing is intuition."

Some clinicians with great intuitive skills are unable to transmit those skills to others and, consequently, are not good teachers. Similarly, when asked to explain how they arrived at some brilliant diagnostic or therapeutic result, they may advance an explanation that they believe to be true, but that actually has no basis in fact. Others come closer to the truth when they state that their reasoning was based on the recollection of a similar case. This is actually the explanation of the phenomenon. The clinicians are not able to recognize consciously what the cue is, but despite this, they respond to it appropriately because the response to the cue has for some time resided in their store of long-term memory.

The clinician acquires such a store of unconscious memories by talking to and examining large numbers of patients. A physician with an excessively busy practice may have to limit the contact with each patient to such a degree that he fails to accumulate such a store. On the other hand, a physician with too small a practice cannot see enough examples of different diseases for this purpose.

The clinician becomes familiar with a disease to the point that he notes the differences and similarities of a particular case when compared with others he has observed. The differences may be so subtle that the observer is not able to describe them, but he knows that they are not exactly the same. It is as though the memory preserves the initial case in something like a photo-graphic negative of a familiar scene. With the second case this memory image is unconsciously placed over the features present, and, just as with two similar photographic negatives, attention is drawn to the places where there is a change in one relative to the other.

The same experience is present with the memory of other things such as stories or music. A child who is familiar with a story, for example, will often call attention to slight variations when it is retold even though he does not know it by heart himself. The perception of change is not a quality unique to the sense of sight; changes in sound, taste, smell and temperature are readily noticed also. Comparison of the old and new facts or images is often a subconscious exercise and is likely the way intuition de-velops. The nature of clinical expertise lies with the rapid and efficient establishment of contexts or hypotheses and in this man-ner intuitions gain access to conscious thought. With this back-ground the clinician's skill in caring for the patient follows a sequential pattern (1) the acquisition of knowledge (2) the gaining of experience and (3) the development of judgement.

The Acquisition of Knowledge from the Patient

The clinician's basic requirement is to become well-informed about his patient; the simple acquisition of facts from the patient interviews. The simplicity fades as the interplay of personalities and biologic differences color the signs and symptoms of an illness in a seemingly capricious manner. Some patients maintain an atti-tude of stoicism when ill; other patients bubble with a constant overflow of symptoms unrelated to recognizable diseases. The questioner may have to extract each answer from the close-mouthed patient. The acquiescent patient may give what he thinks the questioner wants, and the verbose, assertive patient may give what he thinks the examiner deserves. Irrelevant interjections may lead the interviewer far afield. A seemingly irrelevant re-mark, on the other hand, may provide the essential clue to the diagnosis. The diagnostician acquires the skill to weave his way through the distortions imposed by his patient's irrational and quixotic behavior. Such a skill assumes immense value when one considers that logical responses are finite, illogical ones infinite.

The diagnostic process touches on the physician's, as well as the patient's qualities. Some physicians unquestionably have a greater capacity for reasoning — both deductive and inductive — than others. Some prefer dogmatic instruction as their intellectual support; believe all, comprehend little. Some are more skeptical and others more imaginative.

The physicians temperament will modify, in a significant manner, the path taken toward the diagnosis. Arriving in a purposeful direct manner at a sound diagnosis depends on the proper weighing and the subtle interplay of a host of intellectual, psychological, moral, and ethical factors. The physician's nature and the patient's personality present obstacles to proper observation. To illustrate the difficulty, W.H. George tells the following story:

At a congress on psychology at Gottingen, during one of the meetings, a man suddenly rushed into the room chased by another with a revolver. After a scuffle in the middle of the room a shot was fired and both men rushed out again about twenty seconds after having entered. Immediately the chairman asked those present to write down an account of what they had seen. Although the observers did not know it at the time, the incident had been previously arranged, rehearsed and photographed. Of the forty reports presented, only one had less than 20 percent mistakes about the principal facts, 14 had from 20 to 40 percent mistakes, and 25 had more than 40 percent mistakes. The most noteworthy feature was that in over half the accounts, 10 percent or more of the details were pure inventions. This poor record was obtained in spite of favorable circumstances, for the whole incident was short and sufficiently striking to arrest attention, the details were immediately written down by people accustomed to scientific observation and no one was himself involved. Experiments of this nature are commonly conducted by psychologists and nearly always produce results of a similar type.

Not only do observers frequently miss seemingly obvious things, but they often invent quite false observations. False observations may be due to illusions, where the senses give wrong information to the mind, or the incomplete and incorrect encoding of information. A curious fallacy of the first type was recorded by the Greek historian, Herodotus: "The water of the stream is luke-warm at early dawn. At the time when the market fills it is much cooler; by noon it has grown quite cold; at this time therefore they water their gardens. As the afternoon advances the coldness goes off, till, about sunset the water is once more lukewarm."

In all probability the water temperature remained constant and the change noticed was due to the difference between the water and the ambient temperature as the latter changed.

To take a clinical example of this "it's not what it seems" phenomenon, consider the evaluation of a patient with anisocoria. Anisocoria may be perceived as either one pupil dilated or the other constricted. If anisocoria is noted with a bright light (a) but becomes less obvious when the light is dimmed (b) then the eye with the larger pupil has a defect in parasympathetic innervation. If anisocoria persists in dim light, then either the eye with the smaller pupil has a defect in sympathetic innervation (c) or the anisocoria is physiologic (d). Ipsilateral ptosis and anhydrosis accompany miosis of sympathetic denervation (Horner's syndrome) and distinguish it from physiologic anisocoria.

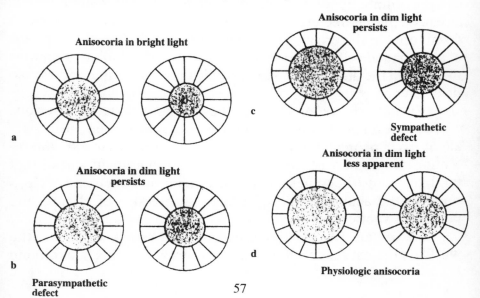

Anisocoria in bright light

Anisocoria in dim light persists

c

Sympathetic defect

a

Anisocoria in dim light persists

Anisocoria in dim light less apparent

d

Physiologic anisocoria

b

Parasympathetic defect

57

Or consider the infantile form of hexosaminidase A deficiency, Tay-Sachs disease. The macula appears cherry red to the observer because the surrounding retina is affected by the widespread deposition of lipid ganglioside. The macula actually is its true color; the remainder of the retina has been blanched.

A clinician must be acutely aware of these medical mirages, these skewed perceptions. Understanding them is paramount in avoiding the diagnostic and therapeutic pitfalls of clinical practice.

Clues and Subtleties

Most diagnoses prove relatively easy to recognize and are no threat to life since they relate to illness that is self-limited, psychosomatic, or without a specific cure. The passage of time often makes the diagnosis either obvious or irrelevant. Many diseases that lead to needless death or preventable disability are seen by the primary care physicians in an ambulatory care setting because the initial symptoms often appear to be minor and the illness rather nebulous and ill-defined. For example, a patient may complain of fatigue, weakness and lethargy. Subsequently, gastrointestinal disturbances may dominate the picture — nausea, constipation alternating with diarrhea, abdominal pain and weight loss may occur. A barium enema to search for a colon malignancy can precipitate hypotension and adrenal crisis in a patient who is already volume-depleted. The diagnosis of Addison's disease is discovered in the crisis. The separation of truly trivial symptoms of a minor and self-limited illness from the early similar symptoms that herald the onset of a major curable disease is a major diagnostic challenge.

Consider the recognition of the insidious onset of a serious correctable disorder whose symptoms are interwoven into a puzzle of psychosomatic complaints. This situation demands the retention of this part of the puzzle and the relinquishment of that until the picture becomes clear. The reading and choosing of clues requires the accumulation of a large storehouse of clinical and personal experience.

Sir Conan Doyle, the creator of Sherlock Holmes, the world's greatest reader of visual clues, drew from his background as a physician to provide the richness and skill that marked his work. Holmes looks at a watch belonging to Dr. Watson and, in a flash, relates the sad history of the downfall of the good doctor's alcoholic brother. He can glance at a stranger hesitating at the entrance to their flat on Baker Street and decide that this is a doctor, just out of military service, recently wounded in Afghanistan. Watson, in his role as the perfect stooge, is always astounded by these visual readings, which always have to be explained by the master.

Holmes' observations are coupled with a great deal of specialized knowledge, he is a student of chemistry, an expert in poisons, he has files of criminal cases, he knows the criminal mind; when he unmasks a clue, in ways impossible for Dr. Watson to comprehend, he is drawing on a vast memory bank of accessible information. We all see with what we know, although few of us are in the class of Conan Doyle's immortal creation, when we are called upon to unveil the meanings of this clue or that.

The methods of Sherlock Holmes are remarkable; they are, clearly enough, the principles and tenets of Dr. Joseph Bell of Edinburgh, expanded and dramatized, applied to specially selected cases of — for the most part — fantastic crime. In them one hears again the dry inflections of the Scottish doctor, laying down his broad rules of diagnosis . . .

"Try to learn the features of a disease or injury, gentlemen, as precisely as you know the features, the gait, the tricks of manner of your most intimate friend. Him, even in a crowd, you can recognize at once. It may be a crowd of men dressed all alike, and each having his full complement of eyes, nose, hair and limbs. In every essential they resemble one another; only in trifles do they differ — and yet, by knowing these trifles well, you make your recognition of your diagnosis with ease. So it is with disease of mind or body or morals. Racial peculiarities, hereditary tricks of manner, accent, occupation or the want of it, education, environment of every kind, by their little trivial impressions gradually mould or carve the individual, and leave finger marks or chisel scores which the expert can detect. The great broad characteristics which at a glance can be recognized as indicative of heart disease or consumption, chronic drunkenness or long-continued loss of blood, are the common property of the veriest tyro in medicine, while to masters of their art there are myriads of signs eloquent and instructive, but which need the educated eye to discover."

Bell's appreciation of Holmes was keen, and his own description of the detective is very adroit. "A shrewd, quick-sighted, inquisitive man, half doctor, half virtuoso, with plenty of spare time, a retentive memory, and perhaps with the best gift of all — the power of unloading the mind of all the burden of trying to remember unnecessary details."

Precepts of Judgement

The case-building strategy of medicine is in effect a process not unlike that used by Mr. Holmes; discarding some findings while adding others until we reach a recognizable syndrome that serves to establish the final hypothesis or presumably correct diagnosis. The process is effective only to the extent that there is knowledge of what information to discard and what information to add and to what purpose. Facts have relative values and experience makes it possible to judge these values as well as apply them to the diagnostic problem.

Experience and judgement mingle together when the diagnostic imperative is a relatively uncommon condition, an uncommon presentation of a common disease or a complication of a disease. Subluxation of the atlantoaxial junction in a patient with rheumatoid arthritis, asphyxia from acute epiglottitis or spontaneous peritonitis in a patient with cirrhosis of the liver demand swift analysis and precise judgement if disability or death are to be avoided.

In acute, as well as less acute circumstances, precise judgement is demanded but may be thrown out of perspective by the peculiar nature of one's own total experience. Fever of unknown origin may present as a case with an array of puzzling symptoms. The specialist in infectious disease is likely to view it as resulting from an infection; the oncologist thinks that a malignancy is the likely cause and the immunologist considers it as a result of a "collagen-vascular" disorder. No one has judgement that is all-inclusive or fully-balanced, but a detached view yields a rational approach to proper evaluation with optimum use of technology and its hardware.

The optimum use of technology is a sequential step that reflects the soundness of judgement. The approach of collecting a reasonable data base as a routine and focusing the search for further information as dictated by sequential hypotheses is not new. Flexner, in his famous report of 1910, compared the clinician's approach to problem solving with that of the scientific investigator:

> The main intellectual tool of the investigator is the working hypothesis. The scientist is confronted by a definite situation, he observes it for the purpose of taking in all the facts. These suggest to him a line of action. He constructs an hypothesis. Upon this he acts, and the practical outcome of this procedure refutes, confirms or modifies his theory. Between theory and fact his mind flies like a shuttle; and theory is helpful and important just to the degree in which it enables him to understand, relate and control the phenomena. This is essentially the technique of research: Wherein is it relevant to bedside practice? The physician too is confronted by a definite situation. He must seize its details, and only powers of observation trained in actual experimentation enable him to do so. The patient's history, condition, symptoms form his data. Thereupon, he too, frames his working hypothesis, now called a diagnosis. It suggests a line of action. Is he right or wrong? Has he actually amassed all the significant facts? Does his working hypothesis properly put them together?

Some clinicians have an instinctive judgement that is as innate to their work as is literary and artistic taste in those who portray a sense of beauty or aesthetic sensibility on canvas, on paper or through music. The one who has such diagnostic and therapeutic taste simply feels in his mind that a particular line of thinking and reasoning is worth following, perhaps without knowing why. The reliability and accuracy of one's feelings can be determined only by the results. The clinician who possesses the flair for choosing profitable lines of inquiry uses his imagination to consider a wide range of possibilities while unconsciously filling in the gaps according to past experience, knowledge and expectations. At the same time, he does not restrict his thinking to established knowledge and the immediate problem. This clinical taste plays an important part in choosing profitable leads to investigate, in recognizing promising clues, in deciding on a course of action where there are few facts with which to reason and in forming an opinion on new findings before the evidence is decisive. The cloud of uncertainty that is a part of complex illness is lessened as the physician develops his powers of observation and acquires this clinical taste.

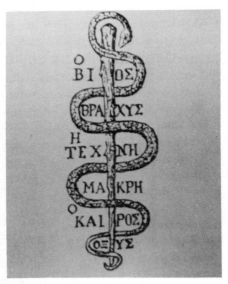

Life is short,
Art is long,
Experience difficult.
(The Aesculapian Wand)

Chapter 5

Mnemonics:

Renal and Gastrointestinal

"(If a physician lives long enough) . . . nothing is more likely that he may find himself fallen under his own reproof and inconveniently confronted by his own maxims."

— Latham

"It has often grieved me to see young men saunter about the hospital square with a little book in their hands grinding a nosology, which they are sure to forget in a few months, instead of going from bed to bed full of interest and alacrity and gathering knowledge which would become their own and remain with them as long as they live."

— Latham

Myoglobinuria

Myoglobin, a heme protein in muscle, stores and facilitates cellular transport of oxygen. Following muscle injury, myoglobin enters the circulation and, in contrast to hemoglobin, is not bound to haptoglobin. Free myoglobin is readily excreted through the kidney at serum concentrations too low to cause plasma discoloration but at urinary levels adequate to impart a burgundy color to the urine. Free hemoglobin, on the other hand, combines with haptoglobin forming a complex which is not easily excreted and which imparts a pink tinge to plasma. This complex is metabolized over several hours, thus clearing the discolored plasma. However, the urine remains reddened as a result of hemoglobinuria and the differentiation from myoglobinuria becomes difficult except by spectroscopy or protein electrophoresis. Recalling the clinical settings in which myoglobinuria occurs is additionally helpful.

Epi-acronym for Recalling the Causes of Myoglobinuria:
Virile — Caesar — Is — Coming
Callously — Crushing — All
Except — Hot — Heroic
Carnal — Elektra*

Virile — Viral illness

Caesar — Seizures (grand mal type)

Is — Ischemia (e.g. occlusion of a limb artery)

Coming — Coma (prolonged)

Callously — Kalemia (Hypokalemia can produce muscle necrosis)

Crushing — Crush injury.

All — Alcohol (alcohol may cause a polymyopathy and biochemical abnormality similar to McArdle's disease — see below)

Except — Exercise (Strenuous exercise, especially when involving the pretibial muscles may lead to a pretibial compression syndrome).

Hot — Heat stroke or hereditary malignant hyperthermia (provoked by prolonged anesthesia and/or succinylcholine)

Heroic — Heroin (also barbiturate overdose or carbon monoxide poisoning).

Carnal — Carnitine palmityl transferase deficiency (or alternatively **McArdle's** syndrome, an inherited lack of muscle phosphorylase making proper utilization of glycogen impossible).

Elektra — Electrical injuries including electrical shock therapy.

Proteinuria

Healthy subjects average a urinary protein excretion in the range of 100mg. per 24 hours, although this may rise to the 300mg. level after strenuous exercise. Trace proteinuria represents a concentration of approximately 5 to 30 mg. per 100ml. This degree of proteinuria is commonly seen in normal individuals and, as an isolated finding, should usually be considered benign.

The word protein comes from the Greek word meaning first or essential. Protamine, the fusion of the words protein and amine, was the name given by Miescher in 1874 for a basic substance he isolated from the sperm of salmon. Protamine insulin, the mixture of insulin with a protein of trout sperm was developed because of its slower and more even absorption compared with pure insulin.

A Long Acrostic for Numerous Causes of Proteinuria:
F-I-S-H   G-L-A-N-D-S   P-R-O-T-A-M-I-N-E*

Fanconi's syndrome — represents an incompetence of the proximal tubule to reabsorb glucose, phosphates, bicarbonate and amino acids. Proteinuria is generally less than 1000 mg per 24 hours and is comprised primarily of small globulins.

Interstitial nephritis — is a potentially reversible, inflammatory lesion of the kidneys caused by a variety of agents (drugs, urate, oxalate, heavy metals). Some features which help to distinguish it from glomerulonephritis are listed in the appendix (p. 211).

Systemic lupus erythematosus — Glomerular inflammatory lesions associated with lupus include mesangial glomerulonephritis (mild proteinuria) focal and segmental glomerulonephritis (usually improves with steroid therapy), diffuse proliferative glomerulonephritis (proteinuria sometimes sufficient to cause nephrotic syndrome) and membranous-type glomerulonephritis (nephrotic syndrome usually without hematuria). Interstitial nephritis occasionally occurs also.

Hypercalcemia or **H**ypercalcuria — or both may lead to deposition of calcium with resultant interstitial nephritis. Hyperparathyroidism, malignancy or any disorder affecting calcium levels may thus cause proteinuria.

Glomerulonephritis — Urinary findings in primary inflammatory glomerular diseases include proteinuria, hematuria, and red blood cell casts. Depending on the severity and etiology, histopathology may reveal glomerular cell proliferation, immunoglobulin and/or complement deposition, and leukocyte infiltration of the glomerular tuft. (For etiologies of the rapidly progressive glomerulonephritis see the mnemonic M-A-L-P-I-G-H-E-'S   p. 72).

Lipoid nephrosis (minimal change disease or nil disease) — accounts for approximately 85 per cent of cases of nephrotic syndrome in children but only 20 per cent of adult cases. Hematuria is usually absent and both creatinine clearance and serum complement levels are normal.

Arterial occlusion (renal artery occlusion). — Patients suffering from complete embolic occlusion of a major branch of the renal artery usually present with acute flank and abdominal pain, fever, leukocytosis, proteinuria and gross or microscopic hematuria. Incomplete occlusion, as in atherosclerotic disease, may produce hypertension and, in a significant minority of patients, is accompanied by a completely normal urinalysis.

Nephrosclerosis — In the patient with essential hypertension, proteinuria occurs usually only after many years of elevated blood pressure. The course of the associated nephrosclerosis varies and cannot be predicted by the severity of the hypertension. In the occasional patient with untreated primary malignant hypertension, however, rapidly progressive renal failure may occur.

Diabetes mellitus — The nodular glomerulosclerosis (Kimmelstiel-Wilson) is specific for diabetes but is less common than diffuse glomerulosclerosis. It has been suggested that when proteinuria in this disease approaches the nephrotic range, the long term survival is less than five years. Other important causes for proteinuria in the diabetic patient include urinary tract infection and papillary necrosis.

Sickle cell — Sickling of erythrocytes in the renal medulla leads to medullary and papillary injury. Like diabetes mellitus, sickle cell disease may cause both nephrotic syndrome and papillary necrosis.

Polycystic kidney disease — may present in infancy, in which case it is associated with other congenital anomalies and a high perinatal mortality. The adult form, a distinctly different disorder, can go undiscovered until middle to late life at which time the patient may present with large palpable kidneys, hematuria, proteinuria or hypertension.

Radiation — Radiotherapy to the abdominal region may produce proteinuria after a latent period of six months or longer. Hematuria is commonly absent, proteinuria is often mild, but anemia, uremia and hypertension are characteristically profound.

Obstructive uropathy — due to urethral, bladder or ureteral obstruction can be associated with renal tubular damage and a concomitant defect in concentrating capacity. Hypertension, however is rarely secondary to this entity unless severe renal scarring has been allowed to occur.

Tumor (benign or malignant) — Urinary tract tumors may be associated with proteinuria. Malignant tumors of the kidney occur most often in children, the most frequent type being nephroblastoma. In adults the most common renal neoplasm is hypernephroma. Other tumors which cause proteinuria include, papillary transitional cell neoplasms and carcinoma of the bladder.

Amyloidosis — is characterized by an infiltration of vital organs with a complex eosinophilic hyaline material. Only 25 per cent of patients with primary amyloid have renal involvement manifested as proteinuria, nephrotic syndrome or occasionally as renal vein thrombosis. Renal involvement is the principal manifestation of amyloidosis secondary to systemic disease such as osteomyelitis, tuberculosis, rheumatoid arthritis and . . .

Multiple myeloma — Renal dysfunction in this, the commonest of plasma cell dyscrasias, also can be due to other complicating factors. For instance, Bence-Jones proteins, hypercalcemia and hyperuricemia may damage tubules. Protein casts may cause tubular obstruction.

Infection — In chronic pyelonephritis the urine sediment usually reveals leukocytes singly or in clumps and occasionally displays erythrocytes. The persistence of hematuria after appropriate treatment should alert the clinician to the possibilities of neoplasms, urinary tract tuberculosis or . . .

Nephrolithiasis — Knowing the composition of a renal stone is vital in identifying underlying causative factors and choosing proper therapy. Calcium oxalate or a mixture of calcium oxalate and apatite make up 75 per cent of kidney stones. Other radiopaque stones include struvite stones (magnesium ammonium phosphate hexahydrate — accounting for 15 per cent of stones) and cystine stones (1 per cent). Almost all radiolucent stones are composed of uric acid.

End stage renal disease — obtained from any etiology is commonly associated with proteinuria.

This list fails to include periarteritis and congestive heart failure.

Reversible Factors that Exacerbate Renal Failure

Acronym: C-H-O-P-I-N in C and D

Congestive heart failure — Excess total body fluid is best removed with diuretics or, in severe circumstances, by dialysis. Digitalis dosage must be modified according to the degree of renal insufficiency.

Hypertension — Depending on etiology, elevated blood pressure should be normalized by diuresis and specific antihypertensive medication.

Obstruction — Urinary tract obstruction can be ruled out by means of intravenous pyelography, retrograde pyelography, and/or ultrasonography. A simple abdominal flat plate radiograph may aid in assessing renal size and excluding radiodense calculi.

Potassium — deficiency leads to a defect in the renal capacity to concentrate urine maximally. Occasionally, associated sodium retention occurs to a degree sufficient to cause edema.

Infection — A urine culture is an essential part of the initial work up of renal failure.

Nephrotoxins — (especially antibiotics such as aminoglycosides and amphotericin).

Calcium excess — much like hypokalemia, is associated with decreased medullary tonicity and an impairment of renal concentrating ability. Prolonged hypercalcemia may result in calcium deposition in the kidney and resultant interstitial nephritis.

Dehydration — Excessive use of diuretics or overly stringent sodium restriction may lead to extracellular fluid volume depletion in patients with depressed renal function. Though severe fluid depletion is easily recognized, modest dehydration presents more subtly and may require salt supplementation as well as a fluid challenge to document.

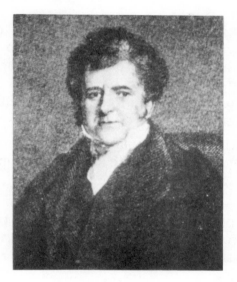

Richard Bright

Acute Renal Failure

In 1827, Richard Bright, then at Guy's Hospital, described "essential nephritis," an entity which for many years bore his name. Bright's disease later became known as post-streptrococcal glomerulonephritis. He is also credited with being the first to distinguish between cardiac and renal "dropsy" by noting that in the latter condition the urine contained a high concentration of albumin.

The causes of acute renal failure, as opposed to pre- and post-renal oliguria can be recalled with the following mnemonic.

Acronym: B-R-I-G-H-T,　T-H-A-T　H-E　W-A-S*

Burns — In severe thermal injury protein rich fluid is lost, leading to volume depletion. Most of this fluid loss occurs within the first 24 hours. During this time, inadequate replacement of volume may cause progression to renal ischemia, oliguria and acute tubular necrosis.

Renal cortical necrosis — is a relatively rare complication of toxemia of pregnancy. It occurs also in postpartum renal failure, which manifests itself one to ten weeks after an uneventful pregnancy.

Infection — Septic shock causes ischemic insult to the kidney and may also activate complement resulting in further adverse circulatory affects. Acute bacterial endocarditis may cause severe diffuse glomerulonephritis whereas subacute bacterial endocarditis may lead to nephrotic syndrome and membranoproliferative glomerulonephritis.

Glomerulonephritis — of noninfectious as well as infectious etiologies may progress on to acute renal failure (see M-A-L-P-I-G-H-E-'S p. 72)

Hypertension — Malignant hypertension, manifested by very high blood pressures, retinal hemorrhages, papilledema, and decreased renal blood flow may lead to fibrinoid necrosis of glomerular arterioles and subsequent acute renal failure.

Transfusion reaction — ABO incompatible blood transfusion causes intravascular hemolysis due to the interaction between surface antigens on donor red blood cells and the recipient's antibodies. Symptoms and signs of such a reaction include restlessness, flushing, tachycardia, tachypnea, back pain, and, in severe cases, shock and renal failure.

Trauma — may cause hypovolemia resulting in renal ischemia. Myoglobinuria due to destruction of striated muscle can also occur. Both processes may contribute to acute renal dysfunction in this setting.

Hemolytic uremic syndrome (and the related disorder TTP — thrombotic thrombocytopenic purpura) — Hemolytic uremic syndrome is encountered most commonly in the pediatric population and is characterized by hemolytic anemia, thrombocytopenia, fever, and renal failure. TTP primarily affects young adults and has clinical features similar to HUS except that neurological manifestations are frequently present in TTP and absent in HUS.

Arteritis (polyarteritis) — Approximately 80 per cent of patients with polyarteritis have evidence of renal involvement. Deterioration in renal function may be rapid and is possible through two mechanisms; vasculitis of medium sized renal arteries and glomerulonephritis.

Thrombosis of renal arteries or veins — Occlusion of a renal artery is usually embolic and produces acute flank pain and microscopic hematuria (greater than 50 per cent of patients). Oliguria occurs only with bilateral occlusion which is rare. Bilateral thombosis of the renal veins usually implies thrombosis of the inferior vena cava and may occur as a result of metastatic disease, abdominal injury or operation, papillary necrosis or amyloidosis.

Heavy metals — such as mercury, lead, arsenic, bismuth, uranium, cadmium, and x-ray contrast media (especially in the dehydrated, diabetic and myeloma patients) are nephrotoxins capable of provoking acute renal failure.

Ethylene glycol — and organic solvents such as carbon tetrachloride may similarly lead to oliguria.

Wegener's granulomatosis — may present a clinical picture similar to polyarteritis nodosa with an indistinguishable renal lesion.

Antibiotics — may induce renal failure by injuring the proximal tubule (e.g. aminoglycoside), by precipitating interstitial nephritis (e.g. cephalosporins) or by promoting serum sickness-like reactions (e.g. penicillin).

Serum sickness — is the prototype of immune complex disease in which circulating antigen-antibody complexes deposit themselves on vascular basement membranes. A list of disorders which may cause immune complex injury and secondary renal failure are listed in the appendix p. 212.

This list fails to include renal failure associated with pancreatitis, Goodpasture's syndrome and uric acid nephropathy.

Causes of Rapidly Progressive Glomerulonephritis

Rapidly progressive glomerulonephritis is a diagnostic term applied to patients with inflammatory glomerular disease which follows an unrelenting course to renal failure and is characterized histologically by widespread glomerular crescent formation.

Marcello Malpighi, one of the founders of the field of histology, clearly delineated the gross microscopic anatomy of the kidney and spleen. We hope you'll excuse our misspelling his name in our creation of a mnemonic for the causes of rapidly progressive glomerulonephritis:

M-A-L-P-I-G-H-E-'S*

Membranoproliferative glomerulonephritis — is seen more commonly in older children than in adults. A wide spectrum of courses occur ranging from asymptomatic hematuria to rapidly progressive glomerulonephritis. Progression to renal failure is the rule.

Acute bacterial endocarditis — especially that form due to staphylococcus aureus can cause a diffuse proliferative glomerulonephritis. If the underlying infection is treated vigorously the progression to severe renal dysfunction may be arrested.

Lupus (SLE) — In systemic lupus erythematosus, diffuse proliferative glomerulonephritis may occur. It frequently progresses to renal failure, though on occasion, high dose steroid therapy has stopped its development.

Polyarteritis nodosa — produces both a vasculitis of medium sized renal arteries and a proliferative glomerulonephritis.

Idiopathic

Goodpasture's — In this autoimmune disorder, antiglomerular basement membrane antibody plays a major role in the pathogenesis of the associated pulmonary hemorrhage and proliferative glomerulonephritis. The combination of pulmonary hemorrhage and glomerulonephritis also occurs in SLE, polyarteritis, cryoglobulinemia, and . . .

Henoch-Shonlein purpura — a generalized vasculitis manifested by gastrointestinal bleeding, purpura in the lower extremities, and arthralgias. Renal involvement, occurring in 40 per cent of patients, is the major factor causing mortality. The syndrome, occurring predominantly in children, generally has a good prognosis, but in adults tends to follow a more fulminant course.

Essential cryoglobulinemia — Cryoglobulins, circulating globulins precipitated by cold, are associated with a wide variety of disorders (especially multiple myeloma and Waldenstrom's macroglobulinemia), but a significant number of cases are idiopathic. Renal involvement occurs in 35 per cent of patients.

Streptococcal infection — Ten to fourteen days following a group A beta-hemolytic streptococcal infection, immune complex mediated glomerulonephitis may ensue. The manifestations of the renal disease vary from mild changes on urinalysis in some patients to severe oliguria in others.

A Passage for Posterity

(A poetic pause for the readers of this nontechnical medical manual)

What an honor it must be
To have a tube named after you,
Like our old friends Fallopius and Eustachius do,
So that passing on, you leave behind something that stuff can keep on passing through.

Access for acqueous
Resides in the canal of Schlemm,
and Wharton has a duct that serves the flow of phlegm.
I get a lump in my sinus of Morgagni
When I sit and think of them.

For me, even part of a tube would do,
Like the ampulla of Abraham Vater,
Or the loop of Friedrich Gustav Jacob
Henle that carries so much water,
Or just some little niche
That some holy fellow hasn't already though a'.

The entrance or exit
To an anatomic tunnel would suffice,
Like the sphincter of Oddi or a
sphincter not quite as nice.

That odious egress upon which all beings human deign to sit.
I've so often been called the same, perhaps I was named after it!

— Robert Bloomfield 1981
(with thanks to Geraldine Zurek)

Hematuria

One investigator has shown that in a twelve hour period up to 500,000 erythrocytes may pass into the urine of a normal individual. Therefore, one to two red blood cells seen in a high powered microscopic field is probably of little significance. The list of the causes for significant hematuria is long and similar to that of proteinuria.

Mnemonic for the Major Causes of Hematuria:
H-E-'S   G-O-T   S-I-C-K   P-L-U-M-B-I-N-G*

Hemophilia — Hematuria may occur without coexisting crisis.

Exercise — (microscopic hematuria).

Shonlein-Henoch purpura — Focal or diffuse proliferative glomerulonephritis may occur.

Goodpasture's — Hemoptysis often precedes or accompanies the onset of glomerulonephritis.

Osler-Weber-Rendu — A hereditary disease with multiple arteriovenous malformations in multiple sites.

Trauma — (often painless hematuria lasting several days).

Sickle cell and other hemoglobinopathies — may have severe hematuria leading to iron deficiency anemia.

Idiopathic thrombocytopenic purpura (also TTP)

Calculi — Hematuria and proteinuria are almost always present.

K (vitamin K deficiency) — essential for synthesis of clotting factors II, VII, IX and X. (2 + 7 = 9 and one more is 10)

Polyarteritis (or alternatively Polycystic kidney disease) — In polyarteritis telescoped urine sediments are often present (RBC's and WBC's and many types of casts). A similar picture may be noted in . .

Lupus (SLE)

Urinary tract infections — gross hematuria may be present in acute cystitis.

Medications — including nephrotoxins and anticoagulants.

Blood pressure elevation — (principally malignant hypertension).

Infarction — (renal artery occlusion or renal vein thrombosis).

Neoplasms — (genitourinary tumors).

Glomerulonephritis — (acute and chronic forms).

This list excludes febrile illnesses which may be associated with transient microscopic hematuria, shistosomiasis and tuberculosis of the urinary tract.

Gastrointestinal section

Blest is the man whose bowels move
And melt with pity for the poor.
He, in time of greatest need,
Shall find the Lord has bowels too.
— Dr. Isaac Watts

Even the ugliest human exteriors may contain the most beautiful viscera.
— J.B.S. Holdane

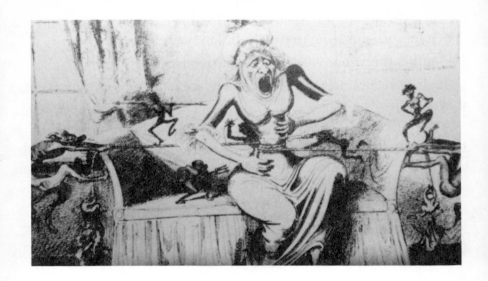

Acute Pancreatitis

The word pancreas is derived from two Greek words which, loosely translated, meant "sweetbread." A more strict translation would be "all edible animal flesh." The organ obtained its name because of its meaty quality.

The word "pabulum," a term related to pancreas and used in the following acronym is defined as "food in a suspension suitable for absorption," "intellectual sustenance," or "an insipid piece of writing."

Acronym for Causes of Acute Pancreatitis:
T-A-S-T-E   P-A-B-U-L-U-M*

<u>T</u>rauma (including intraoperative trauma) — One subclass of this group, pancreatitis following renal transplantation, occurs in 3 per cent of cases and has a 70 per cent mortality.

<u>A</u>zathioprine and <u>A</u>zulfidine

<u>S</u>teroids — Many cases of so-called steroid induced pancreatitis may really represent vasculitic damage from the underlying disorders for which steroids have been given.

<u>T</u>hiazides (and the related sulfonamide drugs).

<u>E</u>thyl alcohol — Alcohol can have a direct toxic effect on the

pancreas. It appears, however, that alcohol intake must continue for several years before the first attack of acute pancreatitis occurs.

Parathyroid excess (and other causes of hypercalcemia) — such as sarcoid and multiple myeloma can produce pancreatitis.

Arteritis (e.g. collagen vascular disorders)

Biliary disease — When a gallstone impacts at the sphincter of Oddi, pancreatitis may develop. If the obstruction is relieved, the pancreatitis resolves more quickly than the pancreatitis associated with a chronic poison such as alcohol.

Uremia

Lipidemias (hyperlipidemias type I and V)

Ulcer perforation (peptic ulcer disease)

Mumps — and other viral infections (e.g. infectious hepatitis and coxsackie B infections) have also been incriminated in the etiology of pancreatitis.

In over 10 per cent of patients the cause of pancreatitis is not apparent. The preceding list fails to include the uncommon hereditary form of pancreatitis associated with aminoaciduria.

Cirrhosis

The origin of the word 'liver' is controversial but many etymologists believe it's related directly to the Latin word for life (and love), "vitalis," or the Anglo-Saxon, "lifer." The imagery suggested in the following acrostic should aid in recalling the disorders associated with cirrhosis of the liver.

Mnemonic: C-H-O-P-P-'D   H-A-M   V-I-T-A-L-S*

Cardiac cirrhosis — is due to right ventricular failure and changes in the liver secondary to hepatic veno-occlusion.

Hemochromatosis — Clinical features of hemochromatosis are diabetes, bronze skin pigmentation, heart disease and cirrhosis. Excessive iron absorption and deposition in organs, such as the liver and pancreas, lead to fibrosis.

Obstruction of extrahepatic bile ducts — is nowadays, an uncommon cause of cirrhosis. Several months of clinically apparent obstructive jaundice is required before irreversible hepatic fibrosis develops.

Primary biliary cirrhosis — differs clinically from extrahepatic biliary obstruction in that abdominal pain is rare in the former and common in the latter disorder. Pathologically, primary biliary cirrhosis affects intrahepatic bile ductules through autoimmune mechanisms, slowly progressing to hepatic decompensation.

Post-necrotic cirrhosis — is found in approximately 10 per cent of cirrhotic patients. Twenty five percent of cases have a history compatible with previous attacks of viral hepatitis; the majority however are idiopathic. Biopsy reveals broad bands of fibrosis interspersed with irregular nodules of intact or regenerating stroma speckled with clusters of mononuclear infiltrate.

Drugs — (e.g. alphamethyldopa, isoniazid)

Hepatolenticular degeneration (Wilson's disease) — the manifestations of this rare inherited condition first appear between the ages of six and twenty five years and are due to excess copper deposition in tissues. Hepatic disease, the commonest form of presentation, is often severe and clinically resembles chronic active hepatitis.

Atresia of bile ducts — Congenital failure of development of part or all of the biliary system will inevitably produce biliary cirrhosis unless surgical correction is feasible and successful.

Mucoviscidosis (cystic fibrosis) — is a hereditary disorder in which viscid mucous obstructs small ducts of many organs, predominantly the pancreas, sweat glands and bronchi. Cirrhosis is secondary to biliary obstruction and is distinctive pathologically, revealing eosinophilic concretions in the bile ductules.

Viral hepatitis — occasionally leads to massive destruction of hepatic lobules and replacement by fibrous tissue. The pattern of cirrhosis is usually of the post-necrotic variety.

Intoxications and Infections — This group includes poisons such as, phosphorus, pyrolidizine alkaloids, amanita phalloides and vinyl chloride. Infections such as brucella, clonorchiasis, shistosomiasis and toxoplasmosis also occasionally lead to cirrhosis.

Thrombosis of hepatic veins (Budd Chiari syndrome) — is an uncommon disorder which may result from local compression of hepatic veins (e.g. neoplasms), as a result of systemic thrombotic disease (e.g. side effect of birth control pills, polycythemia vera) or as an extension of primary endophlebitis. Hepatomegaly with or without abdominal pain and ascites is the usual mode of presentation.

Alpha-l-antitrypsin deficiency — Children who are homozygous for alpha-l-antitrypsin deficiency may develop cirrhosis. In young adults the disorder is manifested predominantly as pulmonary emphysema.

Laennec's cirrhosis — is usually associated with alcoholism, the leading cause of cirrhosis. However, only one chronic drinker out of twelve will develop cirrhosis, suggesting that genetic factors and drinking patterns play important roles (e.g. a spree drinker is less likely to develop cirrhosis). The typical patient has consumed a pint or more of whiskey or its equivalent per day for at least 5 to 10 years.

Sclerosing cholangitis — is a rare inflammatory disease of the extrahepatic biliary tree. It is associated with ulcerative colitis and may precede the bowel disease by several years.

This list does not include glycogen storage disease, a rare etiology for cirrhosis.

Causes of Fecal Leukocytes

White blood cells in diarrheal stool are best revealed by mixing a few drops of methylene blue stain into the fecal specimen and waiting several minutes before examination. With a predominance of polymorphonuclear leukocytes there is an increased likelihood of culturing a pathogen when bacteria are the causative agents.

The causes of fecal leukocytes in a patient with diarrhea can be retrieved by utilizing the acronym, A S-T-U-P-E; a compress of hot liquid and an astringent (e.g. terpentine) which, in older days, was applied by the physician in order to increase circulation to an area.

Mnemonic: A S-T-U-P-E*

<u>A</u>mebiasis — Entamoeba histolytica may invade colonic tissue and cause ulceration which on sigmoidoscopy resembles ulcerative colitis. The majority of hosts, however, are asymptomatic cyst passers. In invasive disease, serological tests (e.g. indirect hemagluttination and latex agglutination) are usually positive.

<u>S</u>higella — a self limited disease, is encountered in the United States mainly among foreign travelers and their contacts. Fever, abdominal pain, and diarrhea containing mucous, RBC's, and PMN's are characteristic. Stool culture is routinely positive.

<u>T</u>yphoid — Salmonella typhi infections occur as a result of ingestion of contaminated food or water. Typical clinical features may include headache, remittent fever, a relative bradycardia, abdominal pain, constipation or diarrhea, a characteristic rash (rose spots), hepatomegaly and splenomegaly. Fecal specimens reveal occult blood and mononuclear leukocytes.

<u>U</u>lcerative colitis — is an idiopathic inflammation of bowel mucosa. It almost always affects the distal colon and rectum but also may involve extracolonic sites, (e.g. uveitis, arthritis, skin rashes). Sigmoidoscopy, the principal means of diagnosis, should be done without prior preparation. Ulcer edges should be swabbed and examined for the trophozoites of amebiasis. Stool cultures to rule out salmonella and shigella infestation should also be performed.

<u>P</u>seudomembranous colitis — Antibiotic-associated colitis may occur with many antibiotics. The incidence is highest with Clindamycin administration but has never occurred with parenterally administered aminoglycosides or vancomycin. The offending organism, clostridium difficile, can be eradicated by discontinuing the responsible antibiotic and giving

oral vancomycin.

E. coli (invasive strains) — Toxigenic strains of E. coli are a major cause of traveler's diarrhea and may present a picture similar to Shigella infections.

Other causes of fecal leukocytes not included in this list are vibrio parahaemolyticus (leading cause of acute diarrheal disease in Japan), lymphogranuloma venereum (associated with rectal stricture and inguinal adenopathy) and Crohn's colitis.

Indications for Surgery in Patients with Inflammatory Bowel Disease

One unfortunate aspect of Crohn's disease is the need for surgery in over two thirds of patients because of fistula formation, obstruction or abscesses. Many will have recurrences requiring a second operation. In contrast, 75 per cent of patient with ulcerative colitis have complete resolution of symptoms, and 15 percent have recurrent rectal bleeding as their only major acute complication. The most important aspect of follow up care in the ulcerative colitis patient is the long term surveillance for colon cancer.

The main indications for surgical intervention in inflammatory bowel disease are recalled with the descriptive acrostic:

I C-H-O-P

Infection — In Crohn's disease, fistula formation can be associated with abscesses and secondary septicemia. In general, internal fistulas unaccompanied by abscesses or other local complications do not require surgery.

Carcinoma — Patients with ulcerative colitis have a ten-fold increase in the incidence of colonic cancer, but those with proctitis alone probably have no more risk of cancer than the general population. After seven to ten years of disease activity, frequent colonoscopy and biopsies aid in determining those at highest risk who may require colectomy.

Hemorrhage — Massive bleeding beyond 24 hours or brisk bleeding that does not respond to high dose steroid therapy are both clear indications for surgery in a patient with ulcerative colitis. Bleeding in Crohn's disease or Crohn's colitis occurs less frequently than in ulcerative colitis. When it does occur, bleeding may be massive due to deep ulceration into a neighboring blood vessel.

Obstruction — Thickened distended bowel in Crohn's disease or ulcerative colitis may look relatively benign on x-ray and yet become the source of frequent partial obstructions with associated crampy abdominal pain. Steady diffuse pain, decreased bowel movements and fever in a patient with ulcerative colitis should alert the clinician to the possibility of acute toxic megacolon.

Perforation — Free perforation, more common in ulcerative colitis, may occur with minimal symptoms in a patient on steroid therapy and requires immediate surgical intervention.

Causes of Colonic Diarrhea

> "And to require the help of medicine, not when a wound has to be cured, or on occasion of an epidemic, but just because by indolence and a habit of life . . . men fill themselves with waters and winds as if their bodies were a marsh, compelling the ingenious sons of Aesclepius to find more names for disease such as flatulence and catarrh, is not this too a disgrace?
> — Plato, *The Republic*

"Catarrh," though it has come to mean nasal discharge, in earlier days was applied in a broader sense to the flow of fluid from any mucous membrane as in gastric catarrh or intestinal catarrh. The Greek term from which "catarrh" is derived meant "a running down" and is found within the word 'cataract,' a waterfall.

A Mnemonic for the Causes of Colonic Catarrh:
Acronym: C-A-T-A-R-A-C-T on 2 I's*

Cathartics — In patients who abuse laxatives for prolonged periods, barium enema may reveal a radiographic appearance suggestive of ulcerative colitis. Sigmoidoscopy will reveal a

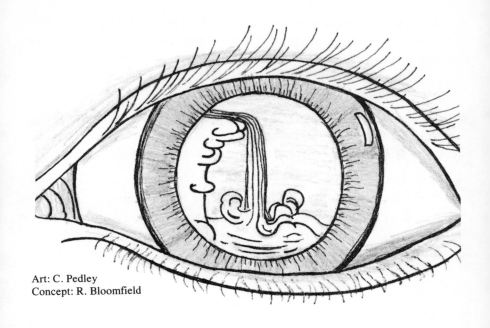

Art: C. Pedley
Concept: R. Bloomfield

normal rectal mucosa, a rare finding in ulcerative colitis.

Allergy — Milk allergy occurs in infants, causing diarrhea associated with stool blood and colonic mucosal inflammation. Removal of milk protein from the diet leads to rapid improvement of the symptoms.

Tumors — a change in a patient's bowel habits in mid to late life, should concern the clinician and prompt a search for carcinoma. A change to persistent diarrhea or persistent constipation is more characteristic than alternating constipation and diarrhea, a pattern more commonly seen in irritable bowel.

Atheromatous disease (ischemic colitis) — Ischemia in the bowel occurs most often in the most distal areas of supply of the superior and inferior mesenteric arteries; the splenic flexure and sigmoid colon. The onset of lower abdominal pain and passage of bright red clots per rectum are generally abrupt and may mimic ulcerative colitis.

Radiation induced enteritis — The bowel may be damaged by 4,500 rads and will almost certainly suffer chronic changes after 6,000 rads. Mucosal damage begins early and leads to diarrhea during the second week of therapy. Diarrhea persisting after treatment suggests radiation-induced vasculitis or ischemic bowel disease which can produce stricture and fibrosis.

<u>A</u>ntibiotic-induced diarrhea — (see pseudomembranous colitis in mnemonic A S-T-U-P-E p. 80).

<u>C</u>olitis — (ulcerative or Crohn's colitis)

<u>T</u>ics (diverticulitis) — The usual patient with uncomplicated diverticulitis complains of constant left lower quadrant pain and fever. Constipation occurs much more frequently than diarrhea. In fact, an older patient with left lower quadrant tenderness and diarrhea is more likely to have carcinoma than diverticulitis.

On 2-I's:

<u>I</u>nfections — causing colonic diarrhea include varieties of food poisoning, travelers diarrhea, amebiasis, tuberculosis and actinomycosis.

<u>I</u>rritable bowel — a functional bowel disorder exasercbated by emotional stress, is often manifested by alternating constipation and diarrhea and associated diffuse abdominal pain. It is a diagnosis of exclusion.

Malabsorption

> Only presidents, editors and people with tape worms have the right to use the editorial "we."
> — Mark Twain

Malabsorption, a feature of certain small bowel disorders, is confirmed by obtaining a 72 hour stool collection with the patient on a standard diet (at least 50g. of fat). Under these circumstances stool fat is normally less than 7 grams per day.

Once steatorrhea is proven a sequence of steps must be taken to determine the etiology.

Mnemonic for the Causes of Malabsorption:
A-S I P-R-E-P A B-O-W-E-L*

<u>A</u>bsorptive surface bypass — (e.g. intestinal resection, gastrocolic fistula, intestinal bypass).

<u>S</u>prue (celiac or tropical) — In celiac disease wheat, rye, oats and barley, all of which contain gluten, lead to villous atrophy and loss of digestive surface area. When the same histologic picture is noted in patients from certain endemic areas (e.g. Puerto Rico, Cuba, Haiti) and the disease is unresponsive to a gluten-free diet but improves with folic acid and tetracycline, the disorder is termed tropical sprue.

<u>I</u>nflammatory bowel disease (Crohn's disease) — Submucosal thickening and fibrosis produce, over time, a rubber hose-like appearance to the distal small bowel in regional enteritis. When there is extensive involvement malabsorption occurs. This is due, in part also, to ileitis which interupts the entero-hepatic circulation of bile salts.

<u>P</u>ancreatic insufficiency — Exocrine pancreatic deficiency occurs in chronic pancreatitis, pancreatic carcinoma and cystic fibrosis.

<u>R</u>adiation enteritis — (see mnemonic C-A-T-A-R-A-C-T on 2-I's p. 82).

<u>E</u>nzyme deficiency — Disaccharidases, such as lactase and sucrase, hydrolyze carbohydrates so that absorption takes place. With a deficiency of these enzymes, unabsorbed complex sugars pull fluid into the intestinal lumen by osmosis and cause symptoms of bloating, cramps, flatulence and, occasionally, diarrhea.

<u>P</u>arasites — (e.g. giardia, strongyloides)

<u>A</u>myloid — Multiple factors play a role in the occasional patient who is found to have malabsorption on the basis of amyloidosis. These factors include mucosal infiltration by amyloid, vascular insufficiency, and bacterial overgrowth in the hypomotile bowel.

<u>B</u>ile salt deficiency — with consequent impaired micelle formation, occurs with cholestyramine administration, parenchymal liver disease, intra or extra-hepatic cholestasis, hypomotility states (e.g. scleroderma and diabetes mellitus) and . . .

<u>O</u>vergrowth of bowel bacteria — as occurs in small bowel obstructions and afferent loops (e.g. gastrojejunostomy).

<u>W</u>hipples disease — is characterized by malabsorption, abdominal pain and arthralgias. It predominantly affects middle-aged men and is diagnosed by demonstrating PAS positive inclusions in macrophages on small bowel biopsy. The disappearance of these bacillary-like forms after long-term treatment with tetracycline correlates with clinical remission.

<u>E</u>ndocrine causes — (Diabetes mellitus, hypoparathyroidism, adrenal insufficiency, hyperthyroidism, Zollinger-Ellison syndrome.

<u>L</u>ymphoma — Intestinal lymphoma may show biopsy features similar to celiac disease but, in contrast to non-tropical sprue, shows no improvement with gluten-free diet administration. Additionally, intestinal lymphoma may be associated with abdominal pain, fever, and signs of intestinal obstruction (rare complications in a patient with celiac disease).

This list lacks some unusual causes of malabsorption such as intestinal lymphangiectasia, eosinophilic enteritis, mastocytosis, Hartnup disease, abetalipoproteinemia and carcinoid syndrome. To prevent mental malabsorption of the preceding material, we suggest reviewing these gastrointestinal mnemonics before proceeding.

Chapter 6

ORGANIZATION

The Literature of Knowledge

> People read, and read, and read, blandly uncon-
> sicous of their effrontery in assuming that they can as-
> similate without any further effort the vital essence
> which the author has breathed into them. They cannot.
> And the proof that they do not is shown all the time in
> their lives. I say that if a man does not spend at least as
> much time in actively and definitely thinking about what
> he has read as he has spent in reading, he is simply insult-
> ing his author. If he does not submit himself to intellec-
> tual and emotional fatigue in classifying the
> communicated ideas, and in emphasizing on his spirit the
> imprint of the communicated emotions — then reading
> with him is a pleasant pastime and nothing else.
>
> Literary Taste
> by Arnold Bennett

The demands of medicine require its practitioners to read books designed to teach them the essentials of their art as well as to enlighten them to share in contemporary thought-life. In a democracy, the average man can take a holiday from thinking only at infinite peril, according to Gerald Johnson. Medical literature spews information, a literature of knowledge, as DeQuincey designates it, that provides the physician with material with which to think. For the physician, as for thoughtful educated persons in general, every age is a crisis and it is informed thinkers, past and contemporary, who interpret the present and illuminate the future.

The professional work of a physician tends to narrow the mind, to limit the point of view and to mark a person unmistakably. On the one hand are the intense, ardent physicians absorbed in their studies and quickly losing interest in everything but the profession, while other faculties and interests wither unused. On the other hand are the "bovine brethren, who think of nothing but the threadmill and the corn." Both are apt to neglect those outside studies that widen their interests, the one from concentration, the other from apathy. Like art, medicine is an exacting mistress, and in the pursuit of excellence a portion of one's spirit may not be left free for other distractions. The intimate personal nature of the physician's work leaves the mind in need of that other education, that higher education of which Plato speaks, — "That education in virtue from youth upwards, which enables a man eagerly to pursue the ideal perfection." For some, the daily rounds and the tasks of medicine furnish more than enough to satisfy their heart's desire, and there seems no room for anything else, but to relish the good company of the great minds of all ages is an all-important thing.

"Personal contact with men of high purpose and character will help a man to make a start — to have the desire, at least, but in its fullness this culture — for that word best expresses it — has to be wrought out by each one for himself. Start at once a bed-side library and spend the last half hour of the day in communion with the saints of humanity. There are great lessons to be learned from Job and from David, from Isaiah and St. Paul. Taught by Shakespeare you may take your intellectual and moral measure with singular precision. Learn to love Epictetus and Marcus Aurelius. Should you be so fortunate as to be born a Platonist, Jowett will introduce you to the great master through whom alone we can think in certain levels, and whose perpetual modernness startles and delights. Montaigne will teach you moderation in all things, and to be "sealed of his tribe" is a special privilege. We have in the profession only a few great literary heroes of the first rank, the friendship and counsel of two of whom you cannot too earnestly seek. Sir Thomas Browne's Religio Medici should be your pocket companion, while from the Breakfast Table Series of Oliver Wendell Holmes you can glean a philosophy of life peculiarly suited to the needs of a physician." So wrote Osler in *The Master Word in Medicine*.

"Every person carries in his head a mental model of the world

— a subjective representation of external reality," writes Alvin Toffler in *Future Shock*. This mental model is, he says, like a giant filing cabinet. It contains a slot for every item of information coming to us. It organizes our knowledge and gives us a place from which to argue."

The physician needs the literature of information to serve as a base for judgement and decisions, for without knowledge he operates in a vacuum, lacking the means even of self-preservation. Physicians are inveterate, nay, compulsive readers and for them critical reading needs no defence, for it is likely to help in understanding human nature and one's total environment.

A considerable amount of background information in understanding human nature may be obtained through careful study of the nineteenth-century novel. The works of Trollope, Thackeray, Bronte and Stendhal portray human nature more accurately than do any current psychiatric texts. Dr. Mark Altschule believes that the medical curriculum urgently needs to have included in it a solid course on the nineteenth-century novel or such a course should be made a prerequisite of admission to medical school, utilizing time in the medical curriculum for advanced studies of the psychological aspects of the novel.

There are rewards from reading the literature of knowledge, but the demands on the reader are rigorous. Such reading requires awareness to discriminate between sound and fallacious reasoning. A disciplined mind that can follow a train of thought to its logical conclusion is required. A zest for living and a noble curiosity about ideas urge the physician forward in his search for the energizing of the dynamic flow of ideas from great books as his analytical and synthetic powers are challenged.

The Quintessence

The first concern of the physician as he reads is comprehension; the quintessence of the piece of writing. What is the focus of the writer's thought? What is the writer's goal or purpose for having laid his hand to this task? The physician grasps the gist of the material as he answers these questions. Grasping the substance is a progressive process, developing as the reader proceeds through the whole body of the material.

Structural Reading

The facility to read structurally develops the physician's sensitivity to the architecture of the writing. Students of rhetoric may use such labels as outline; pattern, design, but all the terms refer to organization — the means by which a chaotic mass of ideas is arranged in a form possessing organic unity. As the reading proceeds the structure, the skeleton, emerges progressively. From the unity of the composition he sees "the long line" emerging. The evidence of superior mentality is seen in the physician reader's ability to visualize a serious composition steadily and completely.

The plodding, word-by-word reader does not read structurally and will fail to see the clear patterns of thought as they unfold. It is the writer's obligation to make such patterns evident, but the critical reader involuntarily, after practice, gets his clue from the writer and uses the pattern of reading best adapted to a particular pattern of writing.

Memory

Acquiring knowledge, its storage and retrieval from memory are basic to the physician's work. Given a deep-seated interest in ideas, grasping the substance of what he reads, noting the outline or pattern of the composition, the physician finds remembering what he reads a logical result. Superficial reading is, however, antagonistic to remembering. If the pattern of thought is encoded in his brain the reader cannot help remembering. The surest way to remember what is read is to read structurally — sensing the orderly unfolding of the author's thought. The physician will recall the substance of a physician author's material and if it is worth remembering will assimilate the author's ideas into the texture of his own thinking and practice. Sometimes by good fortune the actual words of the author are inescapably right and will be remembered with little effort, especially if his style and diction are skillfully employed. Textbook material especially taxes the memory because it is frequently so condensed, and more frequently, the style is so pedestrian that the reader must call on the powers of his imagination to supply concrete instances or specific details to bridge the hiatus between sentences. The burden imposed on the reader by textbook writers is often heavier than necessary. William James' influence was widespread, due in part to his gift of style and picturesque vocabulary. For the dull stuff, the reader must summon his imagination to his aid. In any event as he fuses a body of thought from a writer into an amalgam with his own, he will remember it, for it becomes his creation.

Methods of Organization

It would be unusual to imagine a time that every facet of life was organized to satisfaction. There is always a ragged edge here or a shred there that needs to be made more tidy. Perhaps it is a function of conscience to prod us from our reverie or procrastination to assure a more orderly existence. Parents are surely known to provide the prod from the time of first memory and that stimulus is applied by others as knowledge accumulates. At some particular time, perhaps with maturity, the stimulus comes from within. Some sharpen the skill to a keener edge than others.

The need for applying method to learning was fundamental in the lives of those acclaimed as medicine's greats. Consider Sir William Osler's advice to medical students:

"Given the sacred hunger and proper preliminary training, the student-practitioner requires at least three things with which to stimulate and maintain his education, a notebook, a library, and a quinquennial braindusting. I wish I had time to speak of the value of note-taking. You can do nothing as a student in practice without it. Carry a small notebook which will fit into your waistcoat pocket, and never ask a new patient a question without notebook and pencil in hand. After the examination of a pneumonia case two minutes will suffice to record the essentials in the daily progress. Routine and system when once made a habit, facilitate work, and the busier you are the more time you will have to make observations after examining a patient. Jot a comment at the end of the notes: "clear case," "case illustrating obscurity of symptons," "error in diagnosis," etc. The making of observations, may become the exercise of a jackdaw trick, like the craze which so many of us have to collect articles of all sorts. The study of the cases, the relation they bear to each other and to the cases in literature — here comes in the difficulty. Begin early to make a threefold category — clear cases, doubtful cases, mistakes. And learn to play the game fair, no self-deception, no shrinking from the truth; mercy and consideration for the other man, but none for yourself, upon whom you have to keep an incessant watch. You remember Lincoln's famous mot about the impossibility of fooling all of the people all the time. It does not hold good for the individual who can fool himself to his heart's content all of the time. If necessary, be cruel; use the knife and the cautery to cure the intumescence and moral necrosis which you will feel in the posterior parietal region, in Gall and Spurzheim's centre of self-esteem, where you will find a sore spot after you have made a mistake in diagnosis. It is only by getting your cases grouped in this way that you can make any real progress in your post-collegiate education; only in this way can you gain wisdom with experience. It is a common error to think that the more a doctor sees the greater his experience and the more he knows. No one ever drew a more skilful distinction than Cowper in his oft-quoted lines, which I am never tired of repeating in a medical audience:

> Knowledge and wisdom, far from being one,
> Have oft-times no connexion. Knowledge dwells
> In the heads replete with thoughts of other men;
> Wisdom in minds attentive to their own.
> Knowledge is proud that he has learned so much;
> Wisdom is humble that he knows no more.

What we call sense or wisdom is knowledge, ready for use, made effective, and bears the same relation to knowledge itself that bread does to wheat. The full knowlege of the parts of a steam engine and the theory of its action may be possessed by a man who could not be trusted to pull the lever to its throttle. It is only by collecting data and using them that you can get sense. One of the most delightful sayings of antiquity is the remark of Heraclitus upon his predecessors — that they had much knowledge but no sense — which indicates that the noble old Ephesian had a keen appreciation of their difference; and the distinction, too, is well drawn by Tennyson in the oft-quoted line:

> 'Knowledge comes but wisdom lingers.' ''

Organization takes time, but so does the search for information that you thought you had learned, but cannot remember. It is a skill that deserves the practice required.

Much of life is spent in learning and much that is learned relates in one way or another to things we already know quite a bit about. For this reason a sense of ordiliness already exists, but we may not be aware of it because we spend little time thinking about it.

To do otherwise, to fail to train your memory in an orderly fashion, means that material may be spewed forth in a disjointed manner. Information would thus entangle rather than clarify. The confused state resulting from such jumble would resemble the Watergate story which erupted by bits and pieces, becoming clearer with the addition of each new piece, but never attaining complete clarity.

Clustering information, numbers for example, is a primitive way of organizing material. Scan the number 637405728 and read on. It's not likely that you are able to remember all nine numbers since they exceed the usual capacity of short-term memory. But group them into clusters of three (637) (405) (728), and it becomes much easier than rote.

Clustering organizes numbers for easier retrieval from short-term memory, but it is not an efficient organizational schema for encoding the permanent memory. Clustering numbers of this sort has a weakness that can be overcome; a lack of analysis. No consideration was given to possible relationships within the numbers. For information to gain entry into the long-term memory participation must be more intense, the process more active. Consider the numbers 1, 9, 2, 8, 3, 7, 4, 6, 5. Note the systematic relationship among the numbers. Read on for another page or two without rehearsal and see if you can recall it. This example emphasizes the nature of long-term memory — retrieval without rehearsal.

List retrieval requires an analysis of the list. Can the items to be retrieved be clustered into catagories or is there a logical progression? Consider, for example, a list of toxins that cause bullae formation: blister beetle bites, carbon monoxide, dimethyl sulfate, ethylene oxide, hexachlorobenzene, spider bites, snake bites, trichloroethylene, barbiturates, diphenoxylate, glutethimide, scombroid fish toxins, sulfonamides, tetradon fish toxins and tetracycline.

There is no logical progression of these 15 items. They neither lead from one point to another nor have a logical sequence of order. But, they can be arranged into categories or clusters and such an arrangement reduces the number from fifteen separate items to three clusters: those blisters due to animal toxins, those due to chemicals and those due to medicines.

Now a logical sequence unfolds; chemical toxins with four items, animal next with five and medicines last with six. Undoubtedly a mnemonic would stimulate the initiation of the memory event for a list of such diversity. For the present, we will rest from these considerations and turn to a mnemonic section.

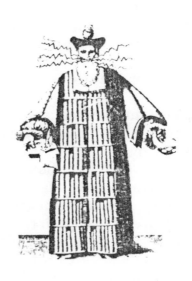

A physician encumbered by his own books.

Chapter 7

Mnemonics:

Cardiovascular and Pulmonary

"I have often remarked that though a physician is sometimes blamed very unjustly, it is quite as common for him to get more credit than he is fairly entitled to, so that he has not, on the whole, any right to complain."

James Jackson, M.D. in
Letters to a Young Physician

"The different medical specialties have one way of glorifying themselves which is common to all. It is by setting forth a vast array of preparatory studies and pretending they are indispensable in order to fit a man for the simple exercise of practical duties that belong to them."

— Latham

Acrostic for the Sounds Near S_2 That May Confuse the Auscultator: P-L-O-P-P-S*

<u>P</u>aradoxical splitting — The most common cause of paradoxical splitting is left bundle branch block. A delayed A_2 also occurs in flow or volume overload of the left ventricle (e.g. aortic stenosis or insufficiency), though these disorders often present with a single S_2.

<u>L</u>ate systolic clicks — are produced by the pulmonic valve in isolated pulmonary stenosis and idiopathic dilatation of the pulmonary artery. An aortic ejection click is heard in congenital aortic stenosis, truncus arteriosus and, occasionally, coarctation of the aorta and aortic aneurysm. In contrast to these, mitral valve prolapse presents with a mid-systolic click and/or a late systolic murmur.

95

Opening snap (O.S.) — A loud O.S. associated with mitral stenosis usually means mitral commissurotomy will be possible. A soft O.S. means valve replacement may be necessary and an O.S. louder than a normal S_2 should alert one to the possibility of a . . .

Pericardial knock (PK) — The interval between S_2 and PK does not change as the patient stands whereas the S_2-O.S. interval widens when the patient assumes the upright posture. PK has an S_3-like quality but comes earlier than the usual S_3.

Pulmonary hypertension — delays P_2 and increases its intensity. On standing, the A_2-P_2 interval stays the same or becomes narrow. An A_2-O.S. interval becomes wider on standing because of a decrease in venous return and a subsequent drop in left atrial pressure.

S_3 — occurs 0.12 to 0.16 seconds after S_2 and is low pitched. A pathologic S_3 is usually accompanied by symptoms of congestive heart failure, but may be present without symptoms in patients with a history of myocardial infarction and resultant ventricular aneurysm.

Mitral Regurgitation

The structures (from right to left) superior to the base of the heart can be remembered by the cue word CAP. These initials stand for Cava, Aorta and Pulmonary artery. CAP also forms part of our original mnemonic for the causes of mitral regurgitation.

The word mitral comes from an ancient word meaning 'cap', 'turban' or 'headband'. It is possibly related to the Greek word for thread or scarf. The left atrioventricular valve received its name because of its resemblance to the headdress of the early Christian bishops — the bishop's mitre.

Mnemonic for the Cause of Mitral Regurgitation:
P-R-I-E-S-T-S'   C-A-P-S*

Papillary muscle dysfunction rupture or fibrosis — Papillary muscle dysfunction may result from ischemia, or from left ventricular dilatation as seen in cardiomyopathies. Approximately 30 percent of patients with myocardial infarcts will develop

96

mitral regurgitation by this mechanism. Rupture of chordae tendinae or of a papillary muscle as a consequence of myocardial infarction or bacterial endocarditis causes acute cardiac decompensation.

Rheumatic heart disease — accounts for approximately 40 percent of cases of mitral insufficiency. Predominant mitral regurgitation of rheumatic etiology occurs more commonly in males whereas corresponding mitral stenosis tends to affect more females.

Idiopathic hypertrophic subaortic stenosis — a hypertrophic cardiomyopathy, is characterized by asymmetric hypertrophy of the interventricular septum. Systolic anterior motion of the mitral valve can be noted on echocardiogram and mitral regurgitation may occur, especially in those cases with an outflow tract gradient.

Endocarditis (infective) — Subacute or acute bacterial endocarditis may lead to mitral regurgitation by involving the valve or chordae tendineae. The 'E' here could alternatively be utilized as a cue for endocardial cushion defects, a group of congenital cardiac disorders including ostium primum defects and common atroventricular canal, both of which are associated with mitral regurgitation.

Systemic lupus erythematosus and another collagen vascular disorder, rheumatoid arthritis, are less frequent causes of mitral regurgitation.

Transposition of the great vessels (corrected) — Corrected transposition is another congenital anomaly associated with mitral regurgitation.

Spondylitis (ankylosing spondylitis) — Three percent of patients with this disease have some degree of aortic regurgitation. Mitral regurgitation occurs with the same frequency.

Calcified mitral annulus — occurs in the elderly and is usually of no hemodynamic consequent unless calcification extends into conducting tissue and causes heart block.

Aneurysm of the left ventrical — may lead to mitral regurgitation due to structural changes in supporting papillary muscles and chordae tendineae.

Prolapsed mitral valve — usually does not produce significant mitral regurgitation. These patients do, however, have an increased incidence of arrhythmias and bacterial endocarditis.

Single papillary muscle — A parachute mitral valve is a congenital lesion in which one papillary muscle sends chordae to the leaflets. Such a mitral valve may be stenotic, regurgitant or may function normally.

This list does not include endocardial fibroelastosis, a restrictive cardiomyopathy seen predominantly in infants.

Congestive Cardiomyopathy

Cardiomyopathies may be classified physiologically into restrictive, hypertrophic, and congestive types. Congestive cardiomyopathy, the most common of the three forms, typically presents with cardiomegaly, elevated left ventricular end diastolic pressures and, in its severer degrees, with elevated left atrial and pulmonary venous pressures leading to symptoms of pulmonary congestion.

Our acrostic for recalling the numerous causes of congestive cardiomyopathy employs the aid of the classic inotrope digitalis. It is hoped the following mnemonic will increase your memory's ejection fraction.

Acrostic for the Causes of Congestive Cardiomyopathy:*
D-I-G-I-T-A-L-I-N,   H-E-L-P!

Diabetes — Small vessel coronary atherosclerosis may be one cause for the development of congestive heart failure in the diabetic, though myocardial infarction is a more common reason.

Ischemic cardiomyopathy — The histologic findings of myocardial degeneration and fibrosis may be due to ischemic injury even in the absence of a previous history or signs of myocardial infarction.

Giant cell arteritis (temporal arteritis) — is an inflammatory disease that affects large and medium sized arteries. Involvement of the coronary arteries may cause ischemia and subsequent myocardial damage.

Infections — may also cause inflammatory damage to the myocardium. Serious viral myocarditis may occur from coxsackie viruses, rubella and echo viruses. Non-viral causes of myocarditis include diphtheria, toxoplasma, aspergillus and Chagas' disease.

Tumor — Carcinomas and lymphomas more commonly cause an infiltrative cardiomyopathy but may occasionally cause a congestive form.

Adriamycin (doxorubicin) — Cardiotoxicity is most apt to develop after cumulative doses above 550 mg per m² of body surface area. Radiation and cyclophosphamide increase the risk of developing this form of cardiomyopathy. Cyclophosphamide alone has also been reported to produce a similar disorder.

Lupus and other collagen-vascular diseases may cause a congestive cardiomyopathy.

Idiopathic — The idiopathic form tends to present in middle-aged individuals.

Neuromuscular disease — In Duchenne's muscular dystrophy, myocardial disease can be detected on the electrocardiogram which shows a tall R wave in lead V_1 and deep Q waves in the limb leads. Other diseases in this class which may lead to a cardiomyopathy include myotonic dystrophy, limb girdle dystrophy, fasciohumeral dystrophy, Friedreich's ataxia and Refsum's disease.

Hereditary forms of congestive cardiomyopathy have an autosomal dominant mode of inheritance with incomplete penetrance and variable expressivity.

Ethyl alcohol in large quantities depresses ventricular performance and causes metabolic derangements which, in time, may lead to permanent myocardial damage.

Lipoidoses — Hurler's syndrome is characterized by dwarfism, mental retardation, deafness and cardiomyopathy. Hunter's syndrome is a similar mucopolysaccharidosis which has a more rampant course with death usually occurring before 10 years of age.

_Pregnancy — Peripartum cardiomyopathy may develop during the last month of pregnancy or as late as five months post partum. Characteristically, the patient is black, over the age of 30 and multiparous. The exact cause is not known though genetic, autoimmune and nutritional factors are felt to play a role.

Causes of Prolonged Q-T Intervals

The length of the Q-T interval varies with the heart rate and the sex of the patient. A table of normal values is given in the appendix. A prolongation of the Q-T interval increases the risk of ventricular arrhythmias and sudden death.

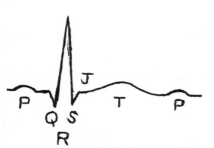

The idiopathic and acquired causes of a prolonged Q-T interval can be remembered by using the letter designations of the electrocardiographic deflections and four H's:

P-Q-R-S-J-T-P   H-H-H-H*

_Procainamide — decreases automaticity, excitability, conduction, velocity, contractility and cardiac output.

Quinidine — is grouped with procainamide and has very similar hemodynamic effects.

_Romano-Ward syndrome — is an autosomal dominant inherited syndrome.

Sporadic prolonged QT interval — is the idiopathic form with no heritable pattern and no associated congenital abnormalities.

Jervall/Lange-Nielsen syndrome — is an autosomal recessive inherited syndrome associated with congenital deafness.

<u>T</u>ricyclic antidepressants — can produce anticholinergic effects (tachycardia, pupillary dilatation), electrocardiographic abnormalities (prolonged P-R, QRS and Q-T intervals and ST-T wave changes), and hypo- as well as hypertension. QRS duration greater than 100 milliseconds suggests serious overdosage.

<u>P</u>henothiazines — prolongs the Q-T interval and may produce transient hypotension by inhibiting pressor reflexes, by blocking adrenergic receptors, and by a direct myocardial depressant action.

<u>H</u>ypokalemia (see mnemonic for causes of hypokalemia p. 43) The other electrocardiographic abnormalities of hypokalemia include flat or inverted T waves, prominent U waves and depressed S-T segments. Common symptoms include weakness, paresthesias, polyuria, polydipsia and nausea.

<u>H</u>ypocalcemia — is usually associated with a normal electrocardiogram except for the occasional occurrence of a prolonged Q-T interval. Symptoms include circumoral paresthesias, carpopedal spasms and positive Chvostek's and Trousseau's signs. Common causes of hypocalcemia include vitamin-D deficiency, acute pancreatitis, renal tubular acidosis, hypoparathyroidism and . . .

<u>H</u>ypomagnesemia — Hypomagnesemia occurs in patients with malabsorption syndromes, in those patients receiving intravenous hyperalimentation, and in chronic alcoholics. Symptoms consists of weakness, tremors, vertigo and convulsions. Severe magnesium depletion is often accompanied by signs and symptoms of associated hypocalcemia.

<u>H</u>ypothermia — produces a characteristic "J" wave on the electrocardiogram. The "J" wave is not specific and may also be seen in central nervous system disorders. In the patient with a temperature below 28-30 C there is a high risk of ventricular fibrillation due to myocardial irritability.

This list fails to include cerebrovascular disease.

Pericarditis

   The Roman physician Galen recognized pericarditis in animals. In *The Taisir,* Avenzoar (1113-1162) first distinguished between a moist and dry type. For the first complete description of the history and physical findings associated with pericarditides, we are most indebted to the physician William Stokes. The acronym we've devised suggests the fibrinous variety of pericarditis. Acronym of for the Causes of Pericarditis:
C-A-R-D-I-U-M   R-I-N-D*

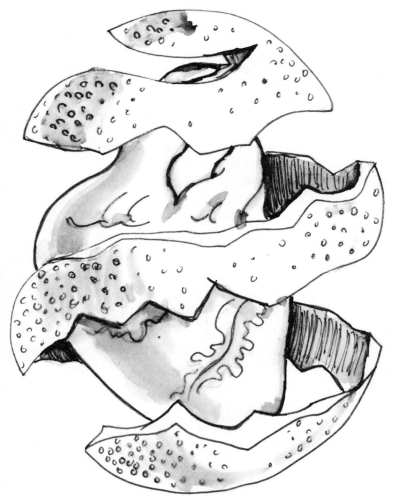

Art: Mary Ingalls
Concept: R. Bloomfield

Collagen vascular diseases — Pericarditis occurs in approximately 50 percent of patients with systemic lupus erythematosus, but tamponade is unusual. Pericarditis is less frequently encountered in rheumatoid arthritis and scleroderma.

Aortic aneurysm — with leakage into pericardial sac may cause pericarditis and cardiac tamponade.

Radiation — Patients who receive radiotherapy to the mediastinal area in excess of 4,000 rads may develop chronic constrictive pericarditis, acute pericarditis or myocarditis.

Drugs — such as hydralazine (by initiating drug-induced lupus), also procainamide and anticoagulants (by producing hemorrhage).

Infections — Viral pericarditis most frequently occurs in young adults, is often associated with pleural effusions and pneumonitis and, in contrast to myocardial infarction, usually presents with fever and precordial pain simultaneously. Other infectious etiologies of pericarditis include tuberculosis, pyogenic bacterial infections, fungal infections, syphilis and parasitic disease.

Uremia — causes a pericarditis which may be fibrinous, serous, or bloody and which responds to frequent dialysis. Pain and tamponade are unusual but a friction rub is commonly heard.

Myocardial infarction — Transmural myocardial infarctions may be accompanied by pericarditis and a friction rub. The pericarditis usually appears 24 to 36 hours after the infarct, is localized and is frequently transient, lasting 3 to 6 days. It is important to distinguish this from extension of the primary infarction and from reinfarction on the EKG.

Rheumatic fever — Pericarditis in acute rheumatic fever is usually associated with pancarditis. Cardiac tamponade almost never occurs.

Injury (trauma) — A penetrating or nonpenetrating injury may result in pericarditis.

Neoplasms — Carcinomas of the lung and breasts, lymphomas and malignant melanomas may extend into the pericardium or may be the source of pericardial metastases. Leukemias may also invade the pericardium causing pain, arrhythmias and occasionally tamponade.

Dressler's syndrome — and post-pericardiotomy syndrome occur approximately 2 to 4 weeks following myocardial infarction or cardiac operation. Common accompanying features include fever, pericarditis, pleuritis, elevated sedimentation rate and arthralgias.

Some rare causes of pericarditis are lacking in this list including, cholesterol pericarditis, familial pericarditis and myxedema (a common cause for pericardial effusion but not for pericarditis).

Causes of Non-cardiogenic Pulmonary Edema

Adult respiratory distress syndrome (ARDS) may result from diverse etiologies. It differs in its pathophysiology from cardiogenic pulmonary disorders in that pulmonary capillary pressures are not elevated in ARDS. Instead, leakage at alveolar-capillary membranes leads to interstitial increases in fluid, inflammatory cells and other blood products. This, in turn, causes collapse of the alveolar spaces and subsequent hypoxemia.

Acronym for Causes of Non-cardiogenic Pulmonary Edema:
C-A-R-D-S, N-O-P-E, I-T'-S A-R-D-S*

Central nervous system disorders — such as head trauma, convulsions, cerebrovascular accidents, or increased intracerebral pressure of any cause.

Aspiration — especially of gastric contents (Mendelson's syndrome).

Respiratory infections — viral and bacterial pneumonia, also fungal pneumonia and pneumocystis.

Drugs — especially overdoses with heroin, methadone, morphine, dextropropoxyphene. Also reported are ethchlorvynol, chlordiazepoxide salicylates, thiazides, dextran, busulfan, bleomycin, cytoxan, barbiturates, nitrofuratoin, and paraquat.

Smoke inhalation and other airborn toxins — e.g. chlorine gas, phosgene, cadmium, CL_2, NH_3.

Near drowning — Salt or fresh water.

Oxygen toxicity — Exposure to greater than 60 percent oxygen for longer than 2 days is likely to produce signs of oxygen toxicity.

Pancreatitis — ARDS occurs frequently in rampant pancreatitis but the causative factors are unclear.

Embolization — either fat embolization or (rarely) pulmonary thromboembolism.

Idiopathic

Transfusion reactions — Leukoagglutination reactions can occur after multiple transfusions. Diagnosis requires the demonstration of antibodies to white cell antigens in the recipient.

Surgery (especially when involving cardiopulmonary bypass).

Altitude — Altitudes above 9,000 feet can bring about pulmonary edema in an unacclimatized individual. Gradual acclimatization prevents development of this syndrome.

Renal failure — Uremia can be associated with diffuse pulmonary infiltrates and some studies support the contention that a substance not cleared by the diseased kidneys can increase the pulmonary capillary permeability.

Diabetic ketoacidosis (rare cause of ARDS) or, alternatively, **D**isseminated intravascular coagulation (DIC).

Shock lung — occurs following hypovolemia as seen in trauma or post-operatively and also in response to bacterial endotoxin.

This list lacks radiation pneumonitis and rapid evacuation of a pneumo- or hydrothorax.

Management of Pulmonary Edema

Whether it is due to cardiac or to non-cardiac etiologies, pulmonary edema is a medical emergency requiring prompt treatment.

Mnemonic for the Management of Pulmonary Edema:
M-O-S-T   D-A-M-P

Morphine — is most useful in cardiogenic pulmonary edema. It decreases cardiac preload by causing venodilatation, exerts a positive inotropic effect, and also serves to reduce anxiety.

Oxygen — Correcting hypoxia is of primary importance in treatment of acute pulmonary edema. If airway collapse is severe, assisted ventilation with continuous positive pressure may be necessary.

Sit patient up — Sitting up reduces pulmonary blood flow and in this way improves symptoms of cardiogenic pulmonary edema.

Tourniquets — Rotating tourniquets also decrease venous return and by this means reduce pulmonary blood flow.

Digitalis — is most effective in cardiogenic pulmonary edema precipitated by supraventricular tachyarrhythmias.

Aminophylline — diminishes bronchoconstriction and augments myocardial contractility. It also may augment myocardial irritability, increasing the risk of ventricular arrhythmias.

Mercurials (diuretics) — Mercurials are outmoded as therapeutic agents, but intravenous furosemide or ethacrynic acid promote rapid diuresis and are effective in reducing pulmonary edema.

Phlebotomy — is rarely indicated in treating cardiogenic pulmonary edema but in severe cases may be utilized to correct hypervolemia.

This classic mnemonic fails to include vasodilator therapy which improves pulmonary edema due to left ventricular failure by reducing cardiac afterload.

Clubbing

Clubbing is usually an asymptomatic finding noticed by the clinician. True clubbing will demonstrate a spongy nail bed, increased bulk in the terminal tuft, increased nail curvature and a reduction of the angle between the nail and the dorsum of the distal phalanx. The main task of the physician is to rule out the possibility of a serious underlying disease.

Acrostic for the Causes of Clubbing:
C-L-U-B-B-E-D   A-I-L-M-E-N-T-S*

Congential heart disease — Cyanotic congential heart lesions with right-to-left shunting cause cyanotic clubbing.

Lung abscess — Chronic lung infections are associated with finger clubbing.

Ulcerative colitis — A stool examination for blood should be done in the patient with clubbing of unknown etiology.

Biliary cirrhosis — Clubbing is also seen in Laennec's cirrhosis.

Bronchiectasis — Other chronic pulmonary conditions, such as diffuse interstitial pneumonitis and the pneumoconioses, occasionally manifest clubbing.

Empyema

Drugs — arsenic and mercury.

Arterial venous shunts — Correction of A-V shunts may correct the clubbing.

Idiopathic — This group includes the hereditary forms which are of no clinical significance.

Leukemia and lymphomas — Chronic myelogenous leukemia and Hodgkin's disease.

Mitral stenosis

Enteritis (regional enteritis) — Other gastrointestinal diseases rarely associated with clubbing include sprue and achalasia.

Neoplasms — especially bronchogenic carcinoma, are the leading causes for clubbing associated with hypertrophic osteoarthropathy. The latter condition is identified by radiographs of the distal ends of the long bones. X-ray findings include periosteal thickening and new bone formation. Cancers of the colon, esophagous, liver, thymus and thyroid have also been associated with clubbing. Metastic disease involving the thorax and pleural tumors are included in this group as well.

Tuberculosis

Subacute bacterial endocarditis — Other manifestations of SBE on examination of the hands include Osler's nodes (erythematous tender subcutaneous papules on the fingertips) splinter hemorrhages under the nails, and Janeway lesions.

This list fails to include the occupational clubbing one may see in jack-hammer operators and the causes of unilateral finger clubbing such as occurs in brachial artery occlusion in which impaired vascular supply to a limb is responsible for the physical abnormality.

The Solitary Pulmonary Nodule

The finding of the solitary pulmonary nodule confronts the clinican with the dilemma of trying, on the one hand, to diagnose a serious disease at a curable stage while, on the other, avoiding overinvasive studies for probable benign disease. A solitary pulmonary nodule is defined as a smooth, round to oval lung lesion which has no accompanying satellite lesions and is surrounded by normally aerated lung. A comparison of particular features which suggest malignant vs. benign disease is given in the appendix, p. 212 An abecedarius for varied etiologies of solitary pulmonary nodules is presented here.

The ABC's of Solitary Pulmonary Nodules:*

A — Artifacts — such as skin lesions, moles, nipples, chest wall lesions, rib lesions, pleural plaques.

B — Benign tumors — make up approximately 5-7 percent of coin lesions. Examples include hamartomas, lipomas, adenomas, and neurofibromas.

C — Cancer — Primary lung cancers constitute the majority of malignant coin lesions. Metastatic disease from breast, bowel or testicular carcinomas comprise less than 10 percent.

D — Dilated bronchus — bronchogenic cysts.

E — Effusion — Interlobar pulmonary effusions may present as a pseudotumor.

F — Fistula — (arteriovenous fistula).

<u>G</u> — Granulomas — constitute another major etiology for solitary pulmonary nodules. Most of these are due to healed tuberculosis. Other causes include histoplasmosis, coccidioidomycosis, sarcoid, and lipoid granulomas.

<u>H</u> — Hematomas — (or alternatively, hydatid cysts).

<u>I</u> — Infection — poorly resolving pneumonias may create a pulmonary parenchymal density indistinguishable from the other etiologies of coin lesions.

<u>J</u> — Joint disease (rheumatoid nodules) — Though most often found in subcutaneous tissue, solitary rheumatoid nodules may occasionally arise in the myocardium, pleura or pulmonary parenchyma.

Pulmonary Hypertension

Pulmonary hypertension can be progressive and unremitting or episodic and completely reversible. The former pattern leads to cor pulmonale and is generally due to persistent hypoxia, chronic pulmonary vascular disease, or progressive interstitial pulmonary fibrosis. An example of the latter variety is resolving pulmonary thromboembolism. The major determinants of pulmonary arterial pressure are the degree of acidosis and airway hypoxia, left atrial pressure, and the size of the pulmonary capillary bed.

Acronym for the Causes of Pulmonary Hypertension:
A   P-U-L-M-O-N-I-C   C-H-O-R-E*

<u>A</u>cidosis — increases pulmonary capillary vasospasm.

<u>P</u>rimary pulmonary hypertension — is an uncommon disease which typically affects young females and pathologically exhibits internal hyperplasia and muscular hypertrophy in the small pulmonary arteries. Raynaud's disease is present in an appreciable number of cases. After definitive diagnosis by angiographic studies, the natural course of the disease commonly leads to death within 5 years.

<u>U</u>pper airway obstruction — may occur chronically as part of the sleep apnea hypersomnolence syndrome. Central apnea and alveolar hyperventilation also occasionally occur in com-

bination with this form of obstruction. Tracheostomy is useful in treating the upper airway obstruction and preventing the associated complications.

Left ventricular failure — over time leads to elevated left atrial pressure which is transmitted to the pulmonary vasculature. Heart failure also causes airway hypoxia and secondary vasospasm.

Mitral stenosis — provokes pulmonary hypertension by the same mechanisms.

Obstructive pulmonary disease (chronic). — Many patients with chronic bronchitis or emphysema never develop cor pulmonale because their disease is limited in extent or is not severe enough to produce the prolonged hypoxia and respiratory acidosis which produce increased pulmonary vascular resistance. During exacerbations of their disease, however, pulmonary hypertension may complicate the clinical course.

Neuromuscular disorders — by causing chronic malfunction of the chest's bellows-like action, can result in hypercapnia, ventilatory depression, acidosis and subsequent pulmonary hypertension.

Interstitial fibrosis — Aside from the primary forms of progressive interstitial disease (e.g. Hamman — Rich syndrome and related disorders), radiation fibrosis, pulmonary asbestosis, sarcoidosis, berylliosis and diffuse lymphangitic spread of carcinoma may cause cor pulmonale. A similar picture can be produced by . . .

Collagen vascular diseases. — Interstitial disease is most commonly observed in scleroderma, though it is also seen in rheumatoid arthritis, polymyositis and Sjogren's syndrome. Systemic lupus erythematosus is occasionally complicated by acute diffuse pneumonitis or acute diffuse hemorrhagic alveolitis. Cases of angiitis leading to pulmonary hypertension have also been reported.

Congenital heart disease — with left to right shunting (e.g. ASD, VSD, PDA, aortopulmonary window, persistent truncus arteriosus) creates high blood flow through the pulmonary circulation. Whether structural changes will ensue in the vasculature will depend on the duration and severity of the congenital anomaly. If present, the degree of pulmonary hypertension may well determine whether or not surgical corrections are advisable.

High altitudes — (chronic mountain sickness). After residing for many years at high altitudes, an individual may develop pulmonary hypertension. Hypoxia and hypoventilation play the key roles in this syndrome. Improvement is obtained by oxygen administration or by relocation to a sea level environment. The decreased respiratory drive in this syndrome is probably similar to that seen in association with . . .

Obesity. — In the so-called Pickwickian patient, how obesity relates to respiratory failure is still not completely clear. Apneic periods and upper airway obstruction are probably instrumental in the development of pulmonary hypertension in these patients.

Respiratory distress syndrome (ARDS). — If the underlying cause of ARDS is reversible and treatable, then the associated pulmonary hypertension will resolve. (For etiologies, see C-A-R-D-S, N-O-P-E, I-T-S, A-R-D-S p. 104).

Emboli — Multiple pulmonary thromboemboli will, over months to years lead to widespread vascular occlusion and pulmonary hypertension. Nuclear lung scanning or pulmonary angiography will provide the evidence needed for diagnosis.

Gross Hemoptysis

Gross hemoptysis, defined as greater than several tablespoons at one time, must be distinguished from nasopharyngeal and gastrointestinal bleeding. Some features which help differentiate these separate sources of bleeding are listed in the appendix. Together, chronic bronchitis and bronchiectasis account for the majority of cases of true hemoptysis. The etiology of the remaining cases is divided among tuberculosis, pneumonia, and vascular disorders. Five to 15 percent of cases remain undiagnosed.

Abecedarius for the Causes of Gross Hemoptysis:
4A's, 4B's, 4C's*

A — Abscess. Patients with lung abscesses generally have purulent sputum, weight loss and x-ray abnormalities.

Arteriovenous malformation (e.g. Osler-Weber-Rendu)

Anticoagulant therapy (e.g. coumadin, heparin)

Aspergilloma of the lung usually presents as hemoptysis and provides a unique appearing roentgenogram with a circular mass surrounded by a crescent of air.

B — Bronchectasis accounts for approximately 30 percent of patients. Most have excess sputum and radiographic abnormalities.

Bleeding disorder (e.g. thrombocytopenia, hemophilia)

Bronchial adenoma classically affects a young healthy female who notes recurrent hemoptysis.

Bronchogenic carcinoma — (15 percent of cases) Metastatic carcinoma is a very rare cause of hemoptysis.

C — Clebsiella pneumonia (exkuse the spelling) and other necrotizing pneumonias may cause gross hemoptysis, but since gross hemoptysis is unusual in pneumonia, the clinician should search for other serious underlying diseases.

Cardiac causes include ventricular failure, mitral stenosis, Eisenmenger's syndrome.

Contusion of the lung. A history of blunt trauma to the thorax is usually obtained.

Cavitary tuberculosis. Hemoptysis results from ulceration of the bronchial mucosa, from erosion into a pulmonary artery or from formation of a mycotic aneurysm (Rasmussen's aneurysm).

This list fails to include Goodpastures syndrome. Bronchitis and pulmonary thromboembolism, while important causes of bleeding from lung, almost never cause gross hemoptysis.

Exudative Effusions

The criteria which distinguish exudates from transudates include a ratio of protein in the effusion to serum protein greater than 0.5, an LDH in the effusion more than 200 I.U., and a ratio of LDH in the effusion to serum LDH which is above 0.6.

The list of causes for exudative pleural effusions is long. So in our demonic, mnemonic mind we have conjured up an imaginary thoracentesis needle; a needle long and flexible enough to pass through multiple anatomic sites, each of which is a clue for one of the many etiologies. Admittedly, we may have gone a bit too far with this one.

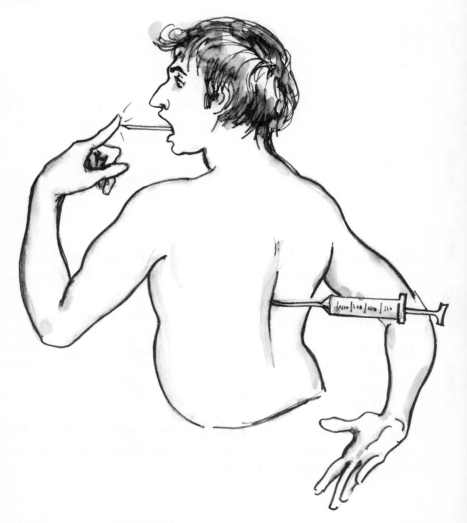

Skin
Systemic lupus erythematosus: and other collagen vascular disorders such as rheumatoid arthritis. Rheumatoid effusions are characterized by low glucoses, high LDH levels and giant multinucleated cells. In SLE pleuritic pain is common.

Fascia
Fungal infection: Such as actinomycosis, histoplasmosis, coccidioidomycosis.

Muscle
Metastatic disease: Effusions in this situation are often bilateral and parenchymal lesions are commonly seen on x-ray. Carcinomas responsible for such effusions include lung, breast, ovary, pancreas, uterus, kidney and testicular cancers.

Parietal Pleura
Post-cardiotomy syndrome: Is associated with fever and pericarditis. Post myocardial infarction syndrome presents similarly.

Pleural Space
Pancreatitis: The effusion is usually left sided and may have an amylase level higher than that noted in the serum.

Visceral Pleura
Viral pneumonia: Commonly causes pleuritic pain but effusions are unusual. They may be transudates or exudates when they do occur.

Lung
Lymphoma: Pulmonary infiltrates and effusions occur occasionally in Hodgkin's and non-Hodgkin's lymphomas. The clinician must consider the other possibilities (infection, radiation or chemotherapy) in this setting.

Interstitium
Infarct of lung: The effusion after pulmonary infarction is usually small, bloody and accompanied by pleuritic pain and scanty hemoptysis.

Alveoli
Asbestosis: (or alternatively **A**bdominal surgery). Asbestosis may cause diffuse interstitial disease (especially in the lower lobes), calcified pleural plaques, and recurrent effusions. There is a relation between asbestosis and the development of malignant mesotheliomas and carcinomas of the lung.

Bronchioles
Bronchogenic carcinoma: (also small cell, large cell and adenocarcinomas) Malignant effusions occur in 15 percent of patients and may be due to lymphatic obstruction or pleural implantation. Transudates are not uncommon in this setting.

Bronchus
Bacterial pneumonia: Sterile effusions in bacterial pneumonia must be differentiated from empyema. In healthy patients, empyema complicates staphylococcal pneumonia most frequently. In those with underlying illnesses, gram-negative organisms such as E. coli and Bacteroides predominate as etiologic agents.

Trachea
Tuberculosis: A parenchymal focus of tuberculosis may erode the visceral pleura, initiating an inflammatory reaction which causes pleuritic pain. The effusion is usually smear-negative and even cultures for tuberculosis are only positive in 20 percent of cases. Percutaneous pleural biopsy may reveal granulomata and provide strong evidence for the mycobacterial infection.

Larynx
ymphatic obstruction: (aside from metastatic disease) This group includes congenital abnormalities of the lymphatics and chylothorax secondary to trauma.

Pharynx
olyarteritis: Pericarditis and pleuritis with or without effusions are common in this disorder.

Mouth
edications: Drug hypersensitivity e.g. nitrofurantoin and methysergide.

This memory device excludes, subphrenic abscesses, uremia and radiation exposure, other causes of pleural exudates.

Chapter 8

Mediation, Imagery and Mnemonics

For the most part, the information that doctors wish to retain and need to recall is comprised of the signs and symptoms of disease, lists, bits of information, numbers, the sequence of procedures to be performed and equipment to be operated. The significance of observation in the search for clues and the arrangement of material in an orderly sequence have been emphasized. The importance of careful listening is obvious. There is, however, something more to the process as we consider association in the role of mediation, imagery and mnemonics.

Association

Association of one fact with another is a fundamental requirement to easy recall. Aristotle defined the primary laws of association. First, the law of resemblance or similarity states that one impression brings to mind another which resembles it in some way. Second is the law of contrast or opposites, which says that where there are two or more opposing impressions, the presence of one will tend to recall the others. And, finally there is the law of contiguity or togetherness. If two or more impressions occur at the same time, or follow closely on one another in either time or space, thinking of one will recall the other.

Similarly, Aristotle penned the secondary laws of association; recency, frequency and vividness. Recency means that we tend to recall associations made recently much better than those made months or years ago. Frequency signifies that the more often you repeat an association, the easier it will be to recall. An association made vivid or graphic through the use of imagery can be recalled more surely and quickly.

Mediation

Mediation is a technique that bridges memory gaps by forming words, connections between words or sentences from isolated facts, numbers and textbook material. The newly-formed word or sentence functions by building a word association which renders verbal sense out of a word that alone is difficult to recall.

Association imposes an orderliness onto the relationship of one item to another. Mediation and imagery, to achieve a similar effect, organize by repositioning information into a logical sequence or orderly fashion. Mnemonics, on the other hand, imposes order using schemas or plans of organization that have been devised and practiced even before the specific material to be memorized has been seen. Often the mnemonic will employ mediation or imagery and sometimes even a combination of the two. A mnemonic is analogous to a pegboard in a workshop, used to organize tools. Within certain limits the pegboard can be used to organize anything, without designating specific places for specific items.

In the practice of medicine mediation can be used quite often to learn lists of symptoms of a particular syndrome or a list of diseases in the differential diagnosis of a finding as in the example that follows.

Behcet's syndrome, a disorder thought to involve delayed hypersensitivity, is most likely to affect those 20-30 years of age. The course of this disorder is variable; usually it is chronic and recurrent but it may be fatal, particularly if there are neurologic or pulmonary complications.

The Manifestations of B-E-H-C-E-T-S

Blood — Hypergammaglobulinemia.

Eyes — Chronic recurrent iritis with hypopyon occasionally progressing to blindness. Lesions occur in about 40 percent of cases.

Hydrarthrosis — Recurrent arthralgias.

CNS — Cranial nerve disturbance, delirium, brain-stem lesions, encephalitis.

Epithelial ulcers — Oral lesions are usually multiple. Recurrent, discrete ulcers on any mucosal site are frequently the initial sign for some time (present in 90-100 percent of cases). Ulcers on genital mucosa will be found in about 75 percent of cases.

Thrombophlebitis — Migratory.

Skin lesions — Pyoderma, cutaneous and subcutaneous nodules and ulcers are found in up to 85 percent of cases.

With practice, the first letter of each symptom or each catagory in differential diagnosis can be used to mediate the recall of the disease in question. The differential diagnosis of pain in the right side of the abdomen can be recalled through the mediator:

T-A-C-T-I-C-S   P-A-I-N   M-O-D-E-R-A-T-E

Torsion of ovarian cyst.

Acute appendicitis.

Cholecystitis or chest infection in children.

Tabetic crisis.

Ileitis — Crohn's disease.

Coronary thrombosis.

Salpingitis, shingles.

Perforation — Duodenum, salpinx or ovarian follicle.

Artery thrombosis or embolus — in the mesenteric system.

Infection in the urinary tract.

Neoplasm — Cecum, right colon, appendix, ileum or alternatively, **N**eurosis.

Mesenteric or iliac adenitis.

Obstruction of intestine.

Diabetic acidosis.

Enterocolitis or alternatively **E**ar-otitis media in children.

Renal colic.

Acute pancreatitis.

Trauma.

Ectopic pregnancy.

Numbers

Remembering numbers is regarded by memory experts as the toughest challenge in the art of memory training. Making notes and keeping files of numbers enhances their recall and a system such as we are about to examine can be effective only if it is memorized.

The most enduring and popular method for recalling numbers is the method of substituting letters of the alphabet for numbers one through ten. There are only ten basic sounds to the consonants in the English alphabet and this system groups sound-alike letters together, while the vowels A E I O U Y and the letters W and H are omitted.

The number one is represented by the letter T, pronounced "tuh" and the association between one and T is recalled because each is written with one downstroke. Number two is represented by the letter N, pronounced "nuh" and the association recalled because each is written with two downstrokes. The letter M, pronounced "muh," represents number three and is associated through the three downstrokes of each. The trilled sound of R, pronounced "rruh," represents number four, associated through the r on the end of four. L, pronounced "luh," is the substitute letter for number five. This association is recalled by holding the hand with the four fingers together with the thumb extended to form the letter L. The letter substitute for number six is a combination, J, pronounced "juh" as well as Ch. The association between 6 and J can be recalled by considering the similarity between J and a reversed 6. K, pronounced "kuh," is the sound for number seven and just as K follows J, seven follows six. The sound of "fuh" representing f stands for eight. F written in script has two loops like an 8. Nine is represented by a "puh" or "buh" sound representing the letters P and B respectively. 9 is the mirror image of P, thus forming an association. The tenth sound is Z or S and is used to represent zero. The association is obvious.

This alphabet comprises the ten basic sounds, but letters other than those mentioned are to be added to the schema because of the similarity in sound between them. Q, for example, is pronounced like K and is represented by the number seven. Although the letter d is a bit dull in comparison to T, there is similarity enough to group them together under the letter one. Similarly, the letters V and F sound alike, as in Fan and Van, and are grouped under the number eight. The Z sound for zero is similar to s as in rose. Thus, the sounds zzzz or sss represent zero.

It is the sound when spoken rather than the appearance when written that indicates the categories of the remaining letters. The first of these is the letter C, a hard C as in Cat, that sounds like K and is consequently grouped under number seven. On the other hand, the C of Ceiling, soft like an S, is represented under zero. The soft G of German sounds like J and is represented under six. The G sound of Gun, however, is harsh, like a K and is associated under number seven. The letter X is in a special category because it has two sounds. There is first a K or "kuh" sound, represented by the number seven and next, the sound of S represented by zero. In transposing this sound into numbers we use those corresponding parts of the alphabet 7-0.

Four sounds remain. First is the diphthong th, pronounced "thuh" as in "that thing" and represented under number one. Second is the ending ng of the present participle, as in walking or talking, represented under number seven because of its similarity to the letter G. Third is the sound Ch as in church. This is pronounced "jerch", sounds like a J and is represented under number six. The last sound is an F sound, as when the words phone or laugh are pronounced. This sound is represented under the number eight.

The phonetic alphabet is mastered with practice, easily taken from those moments of idleness that each of us has. Once memorized, the system can be used to recall long numbers. In the process of practice, however, it is useful to transpose words into numbers, as well as numbers into words to develop accuracy as well as speed.

These ten sounds and representative numbers can be displayed together for easier reference.

LETTER SOUND		MEDIATOR
1.	T, D, or TH —	The Time of Day
2.	N	
3.	M	
4.	R	
5.	L	
6.	J, CH, Soft G, SH, DG, TCH —	Just Charlie and George Should Catch a Badger.
7.	K, Hard C, Hard G, Q, NG —	Karl Caught Gertrude Quickly Walking
8.	F, V, or PH —	Fruits, Vegetables or Pheasant
9.	P or B —	Peanut Butter
0.	Z, Soft C, or S. —	Zeros Circle the Stars

ELIMINATE — A E I O U and the letters W H Y, except H when it is used in conjunction with one of the sounds.

Relating the phonetic alphabet to anatomical parts has been found useful in the process of learning and recall:

NUMBER	LETTER	ANATOMY
1	T or D	Toe
2	N	Nose
3	M	Mouth
4	R	Rib
5	L	Leg
6	J	Jaw
7	K	Kidney
8	F	Foot
9	P or B	A Pat on the Back
0	Z or S	Scrotum or Zygoma

Our first example clearly shows the advantage and ease of remembering a long number with the phonetic alphabet. Consider the difficulty of committing such a long number to memory. 9185271952163909212. Substituting letters for numbers we get B T fLNKdBLNdJMPS PNddN. With imaginative clustering and the use of vowels and W we form this sentence. A Beautiful Naked Blond Jumps Up and Down.

The next example uses the phonetic alphabet in recalling a formula which is comprised of numbers as well as letters.

Formula For Determining Alveolar Oxygen Tension

Pneuemonia, gastric acid aspiration, and atelectasis are potential pulmonary complications in any patient who is comatose, and comatose patients overdosed with narcotics or glutethemide may develop pulmonary edema. The physical examination of the lungs and chest roentgenograms are frequently difficult to execute and interpret in such patients. Arterial blood gases may suggest that one of the above complications is present, but cannot indicate precisely which abnormality, since each may cause arterial hypoxemia owing to intrapulmonary right-to-left shunting of venous blood. A pulmonary complication is suspected if the arterial hypoxemia is more severe than could be accounted for by the hypoventilation and resulting hypercapnia alone. One first estimates the alveolar oxygen tension by means of the alveolar air equation:

$$PAO_2 = FIO_2 (Pb - PH_2O) - 1.2\,PaCO_2$$
Where:
    PAO_2 = Alveolar oxygen tension
    FIO_2 = fractional concentration of inspired oxygen
    Pb = barometric pressure
    PH_2O = water vapor pressure
    $PaCO_2$ = arterial carbon dioxide tension

The FIO_2, breathing room air, is 0.21; Pb at sea level is 760 mm Hg (rounded to 750); PH_2O, unless the patient is markedly febrile, is 47 mm Hg (rounded to 50); $PaCO_2$ is obtained from the arterial blood gas analysis: Thus, the alveolar air equation becomes $PAO_2 = 0.21(750\text{-}50) - 1.2(PaCO_2)$. The formula is translated into a more easily recalled guide by using the phonetic alphabet: PAO_2 = SNOT times (Kolas minus Lisa) minus a TON of $PaCO_2$. Reinterpreted: The s becomes O, the N = 2, ignore the O, T is 1, K = 7, ignore another O, L is 5, skip another O, the s is zero. Lisa becomes 50, and ton = 1.2.

Imagery

Direct imagery is often used by physicians in performing procedures in which they mentally picture each step, each piece of equipment required and each person to be involved in helping with the procedure. Imagery is a useful tool for organizing material as well as organizing the steps to a procedure. The need to dramatize or imagine items in exaggerated circumatances was first emphasized on the scrolls of *Ad Herennium,* mentioned in chapter two:

. . . Now Nature herself teaches us what to do. Where we see in everyday life things that are pretty, ordinary, and banal, we generally fail to remember them, because the mind is not being stirred by anything novel or marvelous. But if we see or hear something exceptionally base, dishonorable, unusual, great, unbelievable, or ridiculous, that we are likely to remember for a long time. Accordingly, things immediate to our eye or ear we commonly forget; incidents of our childhood we often remember best. Nor could this be so for any other reason than that ordinary things easily slip from the memory while the striking and the novel stay longer in the mind.

There are four basic rules of imagery. The first is the use of Substitution of one item for another to improve the vividness of its imagery. The second rule is Out of Proportions or distorting the image in a disproportionate manner. The third rule is that of Exaggeration and is used in a general sense where the whole image is exaggerated. The fourth rule is the use of Action to enhance the imagery.

Aristotle explained the process in *De Anima:* "The perceptions brought in by the five senses are first treated or worked upon by the faculty of imagination, and it is the images so formed which become the material of the intellectual faculty. Imagination is the intermediary between perception and thought. It is the image-making part of the mind which makes the work of the higher processes of thought possible. Hence the mind never touches without a mental picture. No one could ever learn or understand anything, if he had not the faculty of perception; even when he thinks speculatively, he must have some mental picture with which to think.''

Aristotle went on to say that all men can think because ''It is possible to put things before our eyes, the way those who invent trained-memory techniques teach us to construct images.''

Imagery is understandably more effective and easier to use for objects and actions that are concrete. To learn the technique of a surgical procedure, coronary bypass surgery for example, is a chance to visualize a procedure in a number of ways. On the one hand the student can visualize the steps as though he were embodied in the process, perhaps within the heart itself. The skilled experienced surgeon, on the other hand, is able to visualize the anatomic structures, the flow of events involved as well as the desired end result from the viewpoint of his having performed the procedure many times. Each in his respective way knows the process better if he has visualized it before the surgery begins.

If, to use another example, you are preparing to perform closed pericardiocentesis on a patient and are reviewing the needed equipment. Imagine yourself standing in your house or apartment. Imagine 5 ml and 50 ml syringes in the foyer shaking hands with each other. Next, picture three needles, playing pool in a living room, giving their scores, 14, 18, 20, these being the needle gauges. Underneath this picture is the caption, The Big Three, the needle lengths. In the next room, perhaps the dining room, picture a three-way stopcock with rubber tubing for each opening. The rubber tubing is writhing about with a snake-head at the end of each. In the kitchen, picture a pot on the stove boiling an intracath set, assuring its sterility. In the bedroom imagine two alligators wired together dancing on a bed, to remind you that you need two alligator clamps and connecting wire. In the bathroom, picture an ECG machine washing its hands standing on defibrillation equipment in order to reach the sink.

The method of mediation can be used in a similar way to organize a class of drugs for effective recall of their pertinent similarities and differences, as in the following example.

Beta Blockers

Beta blockers have a great similarity with regard to the indications for prescribing. In spite of subtle differences each of the available drugs can be tried in angina, IHSS, hyperthyroidism, prevention of recurrence of myocardial infarction, systemic hypertension and migraine. The key to their use is titration within the recommended dosage range. If, however, one beta blocker, used properly, is ineffective, another will likewise probably not be effective. Additionally, each of the beta blockers, if discontinued suddenly, can precipitate angina.

There are some differences that may make one beta blocker preferable over another because of less prominent side effects. With regard to pharmacokinetics, there are real differences. First, Timolol is the most potent in vitro in a ratio of 6:1 compared to the others which are equipotent. Second, only Inderal has a quinidine-like local anesthetic membrane stabilizing effect (MSA). Third, it is possible that Inderal does effect a greater tendency to mask hypoglycemia. Fourth, only Inderal has active metabolities. Fifth, in lower dose ranges, Metroprolol (Lopressor) and Atenolol have greater beta-1 cardioselectivity than the other agents, thus minimizing the risk of adverse reactions from beta-2 blockage (in particular bronchoconstriction).

The following mnemonic table aids one in the recall of other important pharmacologic differences among this class of drugs.

Mnemonic: N-A-T-I-L

Naldolol

Atenolol

Timolol

Inderal

Lopressor

| N | A | T | I | L |

excretion:

Nephron →   Timolol   →   Liver
                    20%
½ life   renal   ½ life
long   short
14-24 hrs   3-4 hrs.
                                                 first pass
                                                 metabolism

                    solubility:
Non-Lipid   →   Lipid
not completely   completely
  absorbed   absorbed
doesn't cross   crosses
blood brain barrier   BBB
  (BBB)

Additional Comments

Half-life is not well correlated with duration of drug effect, which may be 12 — 24 hours even with short-acting drugs. First pass metabolism occurs in the hepatic-biotransformation of drugs excreted through the liver (I and L). The amount of drug reaching the systemic circulation may vary as much as twenty-fold between patients. All beta blockers alter the physiologic response to hypoglycemia by blocking the tachycardic response but sweating is not affected by cardioselectives or non-cardioselectives.

Mnemonics

Mnemonics assimilates the principles and practice of mediation and imagery into a category of memory training that has, as we have seen, several different methods, each of which has its proponents, but all of which have proven to be effective.

The use of rooms in a house, as in the previous example, is an example of the receptacle method used by the ancient Greeks to deliver lengthy orations without notes. The receptacle method takes material, the type that physicians use daily, and not only positions it in the order in which it is to be recalled but through the use of imagery emphasizes a keyword in each room that serves to associate what is next.

If, for example, you wish to recall the physical features of Cushing's syndrome with the prevalence of each finding. First, imagine a trunk of blubber in the foyer with the number 88 percent on the front of the trunk. This represents truncal obesity. Moon facies can be visualized in the living room with a woman in the moon wearing a dangling medallion with the number 78 percent to represent both the prevalence of the disease in women as well as the prevalence of moon facies in Cushing's syndrome. Hypertension could be represented in the dining room with a large aneroid manometer reading 160 over 77 percent to represent the prevalence of hypertension. Hirsutism, facial plethora and a buffalo hump can be visualized together in the bedroom by a buffalo with a red-faced, bearded woman's head and the number 70 percent printed on a medallion hanging from the buffalo's neck. The prevalence of each of these is about 70 percent. Abdominal striae and ecchymoses can be visualized in another bedroom by imaging the lower half of a body, accentuating the purple striae on the abdomen and indicating the prevalence with a branding iron that imprints 60 percent on the abdomen. Ecchymotic spots can be shown on the legs and the prevalence shown as the blood coalesces to form the letter 52.

The physical findings in Cushing's syndrome could perhaps more easily be recalled by another method, known as the stack — and — link method. Visualize each finding as you stack one on top of the other, knowing that the lower items have the highest prevalence. A trunk full of blubber with its 88 forms the base, surmounted by a moon medallion with 77, a mercury manometer reading over 160 tagged at a cost of 77 cents. The red faced, hairy, buffalo balances atop showing exaggerated striae imprinted with a 60 branding iron and the ecchymotic legs stand atop the buffalo.

Review

Every physician achieves a level of skill and proficiency after years of study. Those years of study, by necessity, included the review, time after time, of the same material. The process of review is the major process by which information is remembered and methods which are explained in this book cannot be effectively used without reviewing the mediator, the image or the mnemonics with the same determination.

Chapter 9

Mnemonics:

Rheumatology and Dermatology

Thoughts for physicians when confronted by patients with unending complaints:

An aged man whom Abraham hospitably invited to his tent, refused to join him in prayer to the one spiritual God. Learning that he was a fire worshipper, Abraham drove him from his door. That night God appeared to Abraham in a vision and said: "I have borne with that ignorant man for seventy years; could you not have patiently suffered him one night?"

— Talmud

And by patients with chronic disease:

And we can say that there are cases . . . in which the disease accomplishes its course . . . by parts and parcels, many times apparently ending, but always . . . beginning again . . . . Yet upon these terms, I have known those who have passed neither a short nor a useless, nor an unhappy life. I have known those who have gathered up the fragments of their broken health as to make them serve for high and useful purposes and put to shame the fewer and smaller performances of stronger men.

— Latham

Rheumatic Fever

A serious sequel to a relatively benign infection, rheumatic fever follows group A streptococcal pharyngitis with an incidence of approximately 3 per cent. If antibiotic treatment is initiated within a week of the onset of pharyngitis, this complication is preventable 90 per cent of the time. The efficacy of penicillin therapy in this regard drops to 67 per cent if started 2 weeks after the sore throat is noted and is reduced to around 40 per cent if 3 weeks elapse before treatment.

When rheumatic fever does occur, it may be confused with bacterial endocarditis, rheumatoid arthritis, viral myopericarditis, gonococcal arthritis, lupus erythematosus, or serum sickness.

The Jones criteria serve as a helpful guide in substantiating the diagnosis of rheumatic fever.

Mnemonic for Recalling the Major Manifestations of A.R.F. as Denoted by the Jones Criteria:

C-A-N-C-E-R

<u>C</u>arditis — Although patients with carditis frequently lack cardiovascular symptoms, the examiner may note any of the following; new heart murmurs, (most frequently mitral or aortic regurgitation), cardiomegaly, pericardial friction rubs, or signs of congestive heart failure. Electrocardiographic changes, though common, do not by themselves constitute clear evidence of carditis.

<u>A</u>rthritis — The acute migratory polyarthritis in this disease most frequently affects the large joints of the extremities. Onset is abrupt and tends to be more severe in adolescents and young adults than in children. Upon recovery the joints return completely to normal.

<u>N</u>odules — Painless subcutaneous nodules occur over bony prominences especially along the elbows, extensor tendons of feet and hands, the scalp, the patellae and the scapulae.

<u>C</u>horea (Sydenham's chorea, Saint Vitus' dance) — Bizarre, uncoordinated, sudden movements may be the sole manifestation of rheumatic fever, especially in children. Its onset is often delayed, and, perhaps because of divine benevolence, is almost never present at the same time as the polyarthritis.

<u>E</u>rythema marginatum is a nonpruritic, macular, pink rash which occurs mainly on the torso, never on the face. It is evanescent and easily overlooked on physical examination. As with chorea and subcutaneous nodules, erythema marginatum is less

prevalent in affected adults than in children.

These 5 findings constitute the major manifestations of —
Rheumatic Fever

The minor criteria include fever, prolongation of the P-R interval, elevated sedimentation rate, a history of previous rheumatic fever, arthralgias, a positive throat culture for group A streptococcus, and rising streptococcal antibody levels. The combination of two major criteria or one major and two minor criteria in a patient indicates a high probability that rheumatic fever is the correct diagnosis.

Systemic Lupus Erythematosus

A set of criteria is most useful in the diagnosing of those diseases which have nonspecific symptoms and signs and in distinguishing among several disorders which present similarly. Rheumatic diseases, in particular, fall into these categories. A set of conditions which helps substantiate the clinician's suspicion of rheumatoid arthritis is listed in the appendix. The preliminary criteria for SLE are expanded upon here.

In the 1800's, lupus was the name first given to corrosive appearing facial ulcerations seen in, what was thought to be, a variety of herpes. The word means wolf in Latin, and was descriptive of the skin, which appeared as though it has been devoured by an enraged animal.

Acronym for the Criteria in the Classification of SLE:
L-U-P-U-S   S-C-A-R-R-E-D   F-A-C-E*

Leukopenia (and thrombocytopenia) — a white cell count of less than 4,000 per mm^3 on two or more occasions; platelet counts less than 100,000 per mm^3. Leukopenia occurs in about one fifth of patients, but leukocytosis is occasionally seen during episodes of active disease. One third of patients have mild thrombocytopenia whereas severe thrombocytopenia with purpura is uncommon.

Ulcers (oral and pharyngeal) — Asymptomatic mucosal ulcerations occur in 40 per cent of cases and are most common on the hard and soft palate. Tender leg ulcers, like those seen in rheumatoid vasculitis, are also occasionally seen.

Pericarditis and Pleuritis — Pericarditis occurs in about 25 per cent of patients. Tamponade is an unusual complication. Other cardiac manifestations include coronary arteritis with myocardial infarction and verrucous endocarditis. Pleuritis or pleural effusions occur in 40 per cent of patients. The effusions may persist for months following treatment and may reveal LE cells on thoracentesis.

Urinary protein — greater than 3.0 grams per day is typically associated with a diffuse proliferative glomerulonephritis, though a small group of patients with SLE have nephrotic range proteinuria without hematuria. These cases have a renal lesion similar in histology to membranous glomerulonephritis. Mild proteinuria does not necessarily preclude a severe renal lesion.

Sm antigen — is a soluble nuclear antigen almost pathognomonic for SLE. It has poor correlation with disease activity.

Sun sensitivity (photosensitivity) — Unusual dermatologic reactions frequently occur from exposure to sunlight in patients with lupus.

Central nervous system disease — In the absence of uremia or offending toxins, a history of psychosis and/or convulsions may suggest the possiblity of CNS lupus. Other CNS manifestations include memory deficits, pseudotumor cerebri, and headaches. Cranial nerve dysfunction may occur concurrently with neuropsychiatric disturbances.

Arthritis — Joint involvement is the most common manifestation of SLE affecting nearly 85 per cent of patients. This nondeforming arthritis affects peripheral joints in the following order of frequency; proximal interphalangeals, knees, wrists, metacarpophalangeals, ankles, elbows, shoulders, metatarsophalangeals, hips, distal interphalangeals, temporomandibular.

Raynauds phenomenon — is characterized by paroxysmal episodes of pallor and cyanosis in the digits followed by rubor of the affected area. Thumbs and toes are only rarely affected.

Throbbing paresthesias or slight swelling may accompany the recovery phase. About one fifth of patients with SLE display Raynauds phenomenon and occasionally do so many years prior to the overt onset of disease.

RPR positivity — Twenty five per cent of patients display false positive serologic tests for syphilis. There is an association with this finding and the circulating lupus anticoagulant.

Erythrocyte lysis — Hemolytic anemia of the Coombs-positive variety is present in 10 per cent of patients. A normocytic normochromic anemia of chronic disease is found, however, in virtually all patients with active lupus.

Discoid lupus — not uncommonly precedes the development of SLE by several years. Occurring in about 20 per cent of cases, these lesions begin as reddened plaques (frequently on the scalp) and evolve into lesions with central areas of hyperkeratosis and follicular plugging. Atrophic scarring may occur in the older lesions.

FANA (fluorescent anti-nuclear antibodies) — Sensitive tests for measuring antibodies to native DNA have replaced the LE cell preparations of the past. Other forms of humoral antibodies can be detected in SLE, including anti-nuclear ribonucleo-protein (high titers in overlap syndrome), antiribosomal antibodies (increased incidence in patients with severe renal disease) and antigamma globulin 7S and 19S antibodies (Rheumatoid factors associated with cryoglobulinemia).

Alopecia — may be patchy or diffuse and is present in 20 per cent of patients. Hair loss responds to appropriate therapy. Recurrent hair loss may herald the exacerbation of disease activity.

Cellular casts (urinary) — Urinalysis is abnormal in over 50 per cent of patients. Casts may be made of red cells, hemoglobin, granular material, tubular cells, or a mixture of these.

Erythematous facial rash — The classic malar flush is present at the time of diagnosis in approximately half of the cases. This butterfly rash leaves scars upon healing. It must be differentiated from rosacea and seborrheic dermatitis.

Carpal Tunnel Syndrome

Thickening or edema in and around the region of the flexor retinaculum of the anterior wrist causes entrapment of the median nerve. Symptoms may include paresthesias, pain or numbness in the distribution of the median nerve (palmar surface of the thumb and thenar eminence, index finger, second finger and the thenar half of the ring finger). The middle finger displays the greatest sensory deficit. Pain commonly radiates up the forearm and symptoms are often worse at night.

Tapping on the wrist with a percussion hammer over the area of the median nerve may reproduce the pain (Tinel's sign). Sustained flexion at the wrist may also reproduce symptoms (Phalen's sign).

Acrostic for the Disorders Associated with Carpal Tunnel Syndrome:
M-E-D-I-A-N   T-R-A-P*

Myxedema

Edema — such as premenstrual edema. In these and mild cases of other etiologies, splinting of the wrist and diuretic administration may relieve symptoms.

Diabetes

Idiopathic inflammation (or fibrosis) — In a great many cases no obvious cause can be identified.

Amyloid — Deposits of amyloid as a result of primary or secondary amyloidosis (e.g. as in multiple myeloma) may produce carpal tunnel syndrome.

Neoplasm — such as ganglia related to tenosynovial sheaths, lipomata, metastatic tumors, overgrowth of bone (osteophytes).

Trauma (or alternatively **T**uberculosis).

Rheumatoid arthritis — Involvement of the tendon sheaths by granulation tissue in rheumatoid arthritis may lead to median nerve entrapment.

Acromegaly — Excess growth hormone causes hypertrophy of articular cartilage and thickening of the synovium, bursae and tendon sheaths in various joints.

Pregnancy — Changes in tissue turgor may be the reason for the development of carpal tunnel syndrome seen in pregnancy.

Inflammatory Polyarthritides

Almost all noninflammatory polyarticular arthritis is due to osetoarthritis though, on occasion hemophilia, sickle cell disease or myxedema may be causative. The common causes of inflammatory polyarthritis are more numerous than this. A handy method of recalling them is illustrated below.

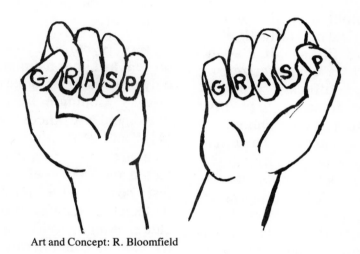

Art and Concept: R. Bloomfield

Mnemonic: G-R-A-S-P, G-R-A-S-P*

G-R-A-S-P

Gout — Polyarticular gout may occur after several bouts of oligoarticular gout. Serum uric acid is often elevated but may be normal. Ninety per cent of patients suffer from classic podagra at some time in the course of their disease but other sites such as ankles, heels, insteps, knees and wrists may be involved.

Rheumatoid arthritis — is a symmetrical polyarthritis often involving PIP's, MCP's and wrists. It is characterized by morning stiffness, predominance in females, a positive rheumatoid factor (about 75 per cent of cases) and a variety of extra-articular manifestations (e.g. pericarditis, cardiac conduction defects, pleural effusions, pulmonary nodules, scleritis, iridocyclitis, vasculitis, peripheral neuropathy.

Ankylosing spondylitis — primarily and progressively affects the joints of the spine and the sacroiliac joints. The hip, knee or shoulder are also involved in 25 per cent of cases. HLA-B27 is present in over 90 per cent of white patients and in 50 per cent of blacks. As in Reiter's disease, young males are principally affected.

G-R-A-S-P*

Gonoccal arthritis — This diagnosis is substantiated by culturing N. gonorrhea from synovial fluid, skin lesions, or blood. Alternatively, the diagnosis may rest upon the demonstration of N. gonorrhea in urethra, cervix, pharynx or anal canal, the presence of pustular, hemorrhagic skin lesions, and improvement through appropriate antibiotic treatment.

Reiters syndrome — may present as either asymmetrical polyarthritis or as uniarticular disease. Common sites of involvement are knees, ankles, MTP and PIP joints. Young men are most frequently affected and 75 per cent of cases test positive for HLA-B27. Associated manifestations include, conjunctivitis, urethritis, balanitis, and keratoderma blenorrhagicum.

Acute hepatitis B arthritis — Arthritis or arthralgias are relatively common in the preicteric phase of hepatitis B infection. Liver function tests are usually abnormal at the time. Urticarial skin lesions frequently accompany the arthritis. Both these and the polyarthritis tend to resolve as the icteric phase develops.

Systemic lupus erythematosus occurs most commonly in women and has a high prevalence in blacks. Nondeforming symmetrical polyarthritis occurs frequently, although often there is joint pain with little or no evidence of acute inflammation. Joint manifestations generally responds promptly to antiinflammatory medication. Renal and central nervous system involvement constitute the greatest threats to patient survival.

Psoriasis — There is a wide spectrum of joint disease associated with psoriasis ranging from sausage digits to erosive arthritis mutilans. The most common form of arthritis is asymmetrical, involving a few peripheral joints particularly the MTP's and PIP's. A spondylitic form milder than that seen in ankylosing spondylitis may also occur.

Scleroderma — Progressive systemic sclerosis affects women two to three times more than men. Predominant clinical features include, Raynaud's phenomenon, sclerodactyly, esophageal dysfunction, pulmonary fibrosis and renal nephrosclerosis. Polyarthralgias involving the fingers, wrists, knees and ankles are frequent. When frank arthritis occurs, its presentation and histologic appearance are similar to rheumatoid arthritis.

Pseudogout — refers to the inflammatory arthritis associated with calcium pyrophosphate crystals in the synovial fluid. Those affected are often elderly and osteoarthritis frequently coexists with this disorder. A uniarticular pattern, particularly involving the knee, is the most common presentation although several large joints may be simultaneously affected.

Low Back Pain

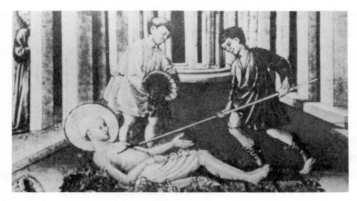

Saint Laurence was forced to lie on a bed of hot coals and thus acquired his high position as the patron Saint of backache sufferers.

The anatomy of the spine, in particular the parts of the vertebrae, was described in detail by the painstaking work of Andreas Vesalius.

Despite his pioneering work in the realm of anatomy, there is not a structure in the body which bears his name. We honor him here with an acrostic for a prevalent malady.

Mnemonic for the Causes of Low Back Pain
O,   V-E-S-A-L-I-U-S*

Osteomyelitis — Vertebral osteomyelitis is rare but may occur following bacteremia or as a result of a spinal procedure (e.g. disc surgery, myelography, lumbar puncture). Low grade fever, tenderness over involved vertebrae and localized muscle spasm are often present. Tuberculous disease occasionally occurs in this region (Pott's disease) and may dissect along fascial planes causing a psoas abscess. O can alternatively stand for Osteoarthritis.

Vertebral fracture — Compression fractures of the spine are seen predominantly in the elderly who have severe osteoporosis. Patients on long term corticosteroid therapy are also at risk for the development of collapsed vertebra.

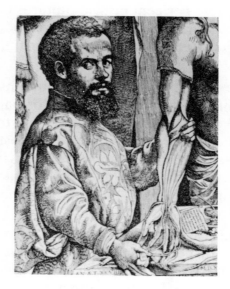

The anatomist Vesalius

<u>E</u>xtraspinal tumors — such as pelvic, large bowel and renal cancers may cause spinal nerve root compression by contiguous spread late in their course.

<u>S</u>pondylolisthesis — a forward subluxation of one vertebral body upon another, usually occurs at L4-5 or L5-S1 and is the result of arthritis or degeneration of the facet joints. A majority of those with this condition complain of low back pain, although sciatica is uncommon.

<u>A</u>nkylosing spondylitis — has its onset in the second or third decade and predominantly affects males (90 per cent of cases). The beginning is often insidious, but over the course of years straightening and immobility of the lumbar spine, kyphosis, loss of height, and decreased chest expansion become obvious. Frequently, the earliest radiographic sign is blurring of the subchondral bony margins of the sacroiliac joints. Syndesmophytes at the anterior and lateral margins between vertebral bodies are helpful in making the diagnosis.

Lumbar disc disease — with aging or disc degeneration, the "shock absorbers" of the vertebral bodies lose their structural integrity and become prone to posteriolateral protrusion. Ninety five per cent of disc ruptures occur in the L4-5 and L5-S1 region. The adjacent nerve roots may be compressed or irritated causing radicular pain, numbness and paresthesias.

Intraspinal tumors — may present with symptoms similar to those seen in herniated discs. Progression of pain or worsening neurological deficits despite conservative treatment should alert the clinician to this possibility. The most common spinal tumor is metastatic carcinoma. (See Kinds-Of-Tumors-Leaping-Promptly-To-Bone p. 8). Also included in this category is multiple myeloma, the most common primary bone tumor of the spine.

Unhappiness (depression, malingering) — The occurrence of multiple somatic complaints, symptoms out of proportion to objective signs of disability, or inconsistencies in symptoms and physical signs will suggest either of these conditions.

Strain (musculoligamentous injury) — The patient often gives a history of injury and either immediate or delayed onset of pain in the lower back with occasional radiation of pain down the buttocks and thighs. A number of related pathological conditions may cause this derangement, including partial ligament tears, muscle insertion tears and muscle hemorrhage.

Signs of Spinal Cord Compression

Spinal cord compression is a neurologic emergency that may be secondary to epidural compression (as in metastatic carcinoma, lymphoma, multiple myeloma, epidural abscess or hematoma), intradural compression (meningioma, neurofibroma) or intramedullary compression (glioma, ependymoma).

The anatomical spine received its name in a round about manner. The Latin word 'spina' simply meant thorn, but spina was also the name applied to the high wall which equally divided the ancient Roman circus, the stadium for chariot races. The wall was adorned with obelisks and statues, giving it a thorny appearance. The back bone's resemblance to this bristling boundary explains the nomenclature.

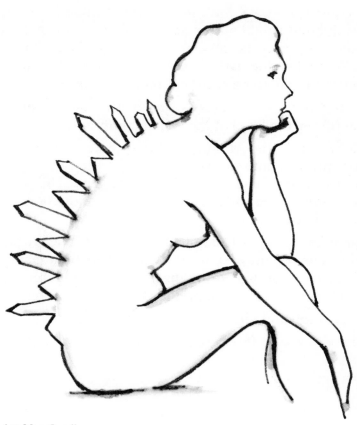

Art: Mary Ingalls
Concept: R. Bloomfield

Acrostic for the Signs of Spinal Compression
S-H-A-R-P W-A-L-L*

<u>S</u>ensory level — A sensory level is not always demonstrable but the physical examination will reveal loss or decreased pin-prick sensation in the lower extremities or torso.

<u>H</u>yperreflexia — Slight hyperreflexia is a frequent early sign of this condition although hyporeflexia may occur in early acute cord compression or if the lesion is at the level of the reflex arc.

Anhydrosis — Decreased sweating below the level of the lesion is an early sign of spinal cord compression.

Retraction of the toes (Babinski) — In acute spinal disorders spinal shock may be present and thus, initially, signs due to disinhibited spinal motor neurons (spasticity, hyperreflexia, Babinskis) may be absent. These signs may take days to weeks to develop in this situation. In more chronic situations they are likely to be seen on first presentation.

Pain over vertebrae — This is one of the most useful signs in identifying the level of the spinal compression.

Weakness — It is important to distinguish neuropathic weakness from primary muscle weakness, as is seen in muscular dystrophy or toxic and metabolic myopathies. The serum CPK, electromyogram and peripheral nerve conduction studies are helpful in this regard.

Anal sphincter laxity — Loss of anal sphincter tone is a late sign of spinal cord compression. Early on, the patient may complain of constipation and of changes in urinary habits (urinating either more or less than previously).

Loss of position and vibration sense (early sign).

Loss of abdominal reflexes (late sign.)

Dermatology

"God will not look you over for medals, degrees or diplomas, but for scars."

— Elbert Hubbard

Nonscarring Alopecia

"A hair in the head is worth two in the brush."

— Oliver Herford

Foremost in the differential diagnoses of alopecia is identifying whether a scarring or non-scarring form is present. In the former, follicles are destroyed and hair regrowth will not occur. In non-scarring alopecia the scalp retains its hair follicles and the hair may regrow. The causes of scarring alopecia include burns, radiation, chronic traction, deep cellulitis, discoid lupus, lichen planus, and cutaneous neoplasms. Alopecia, however, is most often non-scarring. The etiologies are noted below.

Acronym for the Causes of Non-scarring Alopecia
M-A-D   A-S   H-A-T-T-E-R-S*

Male pattern alopecia — is the most common cause of hair loss. It occurs any time following puberty and is related to age, genetic factors, and androgens. Patterns vary among patients and include frontal, temporal, central or vertex alopecia. Females may also be affected but the pattern tends to be central or frontal without complete hair loss in these areas. Advanced alopecia in a woman should prompt a work-up for masculinizing syndromes.

Alopecia areata — is a disorder of unknown etiology with an unpredictable course which is characterized by sharply marginated hair loss in one or several areas of the scalp. The whole scalp may be involved (alopecia totalis) and occasionally the entire body may be affected (alopecia universalis). Finding "exclamation point" hairs, with a shaggy tip and a tapered atrophic bulb, at the periphery of lesions is very suggestive of the diagnosis.

Dermatophyte infections — can involve the beard, eyebrows and eyelashes as well as the scalp. Children are affected most commonly by these infections. The etiologic agents include Microsporum and Trichophyton species. Scaling and prominent follicles are characteristic.

A (hypervitaminosis A) — In infants, the signs of excess vitamin A include drowsiness, vomiting, increased intracranial pressure, failure to thrive, hepatomegaly and alopecia. In adults hypervitaminosis A is accompanied by similar signs but, additionally, calcification of ligaments and tendons, and bone pain may be manifested.

Secondary syphilis — can cause a generally mild alopecia in multiple areas providing a moth-eaten appearance to the scalp. Other dermatologic manifestations of secondary syphilis include a wide variety of skin lesions such as symmetrical red circular papules, scaly brown palmar macules, and, rarely pustules on the palms and soles.

Hypothyroidism — and other hypometabolic states such as hypopituitarism and hypoparathyroidism.

Anticoagulants (and other medications) — Coumadin, heparin methotrexate, cytoxan, colchicine.

Trichotillomania — occurs predominantly in children and adolescents, especially in females. Often one can obtain a history of pulling or rubbing the hair. Morphology serves as the main clue to the cause, with focal areas of thinning, hairs of irregular lengths and oddly shaped bald areas.

Trauma — Hot combs, tight hair rollers, excessive use of bleaching agent or overly vigorous rubbing produces alopecia. Frequently the distribution is bitemporal and hairs will be broken off at various levels. The hair shaft microscopically appears splintered with ends resembling a straw broom. Repeated or severe trauma may produce scarring alopecia.

Effluvium (telogen effluvium) — is a diffuse decrease in hair density brought on by a variety of conditions including stress, surgery, parturition, malnutrition, iron deficiency, high fever, and myocardial infarction. Characteristically, the number of telogen (resting) hairs is greatly increased beyond the normal 20 per cent.

Radiation or electron beam therapy — depending on the dosage, may cause cicatricial or non-cicatricial alopecia.

Systemic lupus erythematosus — Alopecia, generalized and often frontal, is one of the preliminary criteria for making the diagnosis of SLE. (See L-U-P-U-S S-C-A-R-R-E-D F-A-C-E p. 133).

The Plain P's of Lichen Planus

Puzzling — Lichen planus can be mimicked by many skin diseases such as psoriasis, sarcoid, seborrheic dermatitis and drug eruptions (especially from antimalarials).

Polygonal

Purple

Papular — The polygonal purple papules of lichen planus occur most often on the flexor surfaces of the extremities, display minimal scaling, and are often symmetrical and linear. Oral mucosal erosions or hyperkeratosis are frequently present.

Pruritis is often severe.

Persistent — Lichen planus tends to persist for several months but may last as long as several years.

Pigmentation — Discrete areas of hyperpigmentation may occur on the flexor surfaces of extremities, especially on the wrists.

Erythema Nodosum

Bilateral tender erythematous nodules on the anterior aspect of the lower extremities are characteristic of erythema nodosum. The lesions are relatively immobile, often purpuric, only slightly elevated and never ulcerated. Upon resolution, the nodules rarely leave scars or signs of skin atrophy. A similar rash, termed nodular liquefying panniculitis, occurs in association with pancreatic neoplasia and acute pancreatitis. In contrast to erythema nodosum, the nodules in this disorder are always mobile, may develop into bullae-like lesions and may involute to leave slightly depressed hyperpigmented scars.

Acrostic for Diseases Associated with Erythema Nodosum: S-P-L-O-T-C-H-Y   T-I-B-I-A-L-S*

Sarcoid — Although pulmonary involvement is the most frequent and often the most clinically important finding in sarcoid, skin lesions are also common, occurring in about 30 per cent of cases. Various forms of lesions may be seen, including red raised plaques or papules around the eyes, nose and mouth, mucosal lesions, hyper-or hypopigmentation, and erythema nodosum.

Psitticosis — Chlamydia psittaci, a gram negative intracellular organism, is transmitted from birds to humans and causes variable clinical manifestations. Among the most frequent symptoms and signs are fever, headache (often the chief complaint), myalgias, upper respiratory symptoms, (especially a nonproductive cough) and patchy infiltration on radiographs of the lungs. This picture may be easily confused with mycoplasma pneumonia or tuberculosis.

Lupus (SLE) — There is a wide spectrum of cutaneous manifestations associated with SLE including the classic facial butterfly rash, patchy or diffuse alopecia, Raynaud's phenomenon, discoid lupus, and dermal vasculitis. In more than 50 per cent of cases immunofluorescent-bandlike deposition of immunoglobulins at the dermal-epidermal junction can be demonstrated on biopsy of normal appearing skin. There is a greater incidence of this finding in patients with lupus-related renal disease.

Oral contraceptives — It is thought that the progesterone in birth control pills is responsible for the development of erythema nodosum.

Tuberculosis — Dermatologic manifestations of tuberculosis include scrofuloderma (cervical and supraclavicular firm, subcutaneous, painless red nodules), genital ulcers (tender, indurated and associated with adenopathy), livedo reticularis (net-like red or blue mottling of the lower extremities) and erythema nodosum.

Coccidioidomycosis (or alternatively Cat Scratch fever) — Coccidioides immitis is endemic to the Southwestern United States and parts of Argentina. Inhalation of spores generally produces mild or asymptomatic disease. The most frequent symptoms are chest pain and a nonproductive cough. Erythema nodosum, when it occurs, is associated with a benign course. Cat scratch disease is an infectious disease characterized by a papular lesion at the site of innoculation and regional lymphadenitis, which suppurates and drains spontaneously. Both erythema nodosum and erythema multiforme have been reported in this disorder.

Histoplasmosis — Histoplasma capsulatum may give rise to a wide variety of clinical pictures. Possible presentations include a self limited acute pneumonitis, chronic localized pulmonary involvement resembling tuberculosis, mucocutaneous ulcers, and disseminated disease. Erythema nodosum and erythema multiforme have tended to occur most frequently in middle aged women affected by this disease.

Yersinia infections — Y. pseudotuberculosis and Y. enterocolitica have been associated with diarrheal disease, mesenteric adenitis, polyarthritis and erythema nodosum.

Trichophyton infection (and other dermatophytoses).

Iodides and Bromides — may cause skin lesions which usually resemble acneform eruptions but occasionally there are nodular lesions including erythema nodosum.

Blastomycosis (or alternatively **B**ehcet's) — Blastomycosis is a fungal disease acquired by inhalation of spores which disseminate to skin and bone. Most cases occur in Southeastern United States and Mississippi River Valley. Behcet's disease is characterized by recurrent attacks of genital and oral ulceration, ocular involvement (iridocyclitis, uveitis, conjunctivitis, keratitis) and dermatologic manifestations (erythema multiforme, cellulitis, acneform eruptions, or erythema nodosum).

Inflammatory bowel disease (Ulcerative colitis) — Erythema nodosum occurs, on occasion, during the active phase of colitis and is frequently accompanied by the arthralgias or arthritis seen in this disorder.

Arteritis (polyarteritis nodosa) — The organs most frequently involved in this necrotizing and inflammatory disorder include the kidneys, gastrointestinal tract (mesenteric vasculitis) myocardium, pericardium, pleura, and skin (ecchymoses, ulceration, nodules, gangrene).

Lymphogranuloma venereum (or alternatively Leprosy) — Lymphogranuloma venereum, caused by chlamydia trachomatis, is a sexually transmitted disease in which a painless primary gential ulcer or papule is followed by painful inguinal lymphadenitis. Erythema nodosum, erythema multiforme, and urticaria occasionally occur. Erythema nodosum may also be the first sign of lepromatous leprosy or it may occur after initiation of treatment for this granulomatous disease.

Streptococcal infections — Streptococcal pharyngitis is the most common cause of erythema nodosum in the United States. Erythema nodosum may accompany the pharyngitis or may appear as late as three weeks after the onset of infection. In streptococcal sore throat, cough and coryza are typically absent while tonsillar exudate, tender cervical lymphadenopathy and fever are often present. Among children, abdominal pain and nausea may be prominent symptoms.

Diffuse Hyperpigmentation

The color of a healthy person's skin is a result of a combination of many factors; skin thickness, the state of hydration, melanin, carotene, oxyhemoglobin and deoxyhemoglobin. In various disease states, bilirubin elevation also plays an important role in altering the skin's hue.

Two mnemonics are presented here for recalling the numerous causes of diffuse hyperpigmentation.

Mnemonic for the Endocrine Causes of Diffuse Hyperpigmentation:
A-C-T-H*

Although the principal role of ACTH is to stimulate secretion of hydrocortisone from the adrenal gland, it also may be responsible for darkening the skin in certain disorders due to ACTH's melanocyte stimulating hormone-like effect.

Addison's disease — Primary adrenal insufficiency may result from autoimmune disease, infectious diseases such as tuberculosis, histoplasmosis, coccidioidomycosis, and crytococcosis, or metastic disease. Hyperpigmentation of the skin is almost always present and many patients have darkened patches on mucous membranes as well. Areas of vitiligo appear in a small percentage of cases (For the A's of Addison's disease — see mnemonic on p. 13).

Cushing's syndrome — often develops insidiously. The classic symptoms and signs include "moon facies," a "buffalo hump," truncal obesity, fatiguability, hypertension, hirsutism, easy bruisability, amenorrhea and personality changes. Cutaneous striae result from weakening of the dermal collagen fibers. Addisonian hyperpigmentation occurs in Cushing's syndrome only when ACTH levels are increased. This can happen with prolonged exogenous ACTH administration or with . . .

Tumors — Pituitary tumors may produce ACTH. Nonendocrine tumors may secrete ACTH-like or MSH-like substances. Neoplasms in this category include oat cell carcinoma of the lung, bronchogenic carcinoma, thymoma, pancreatic carcinoma and bronchial adenoma.

Hyperthyroidism — Hyperpigmentation of the skin, with or without vitiligo, is not uncommon in hyperthyroidism. Better known dermatologic findings include the raised, thickened, peau d' orange-like pretibial myxedema, temporal alopecia, and the velvety, warm skin of patients with this condition.

Mnemonic for the Causes of Diffuse Hyperpigmentation (non-endocrine and endocrine causes):
P-I-M-P-L-E-D   A-S-S*

Primary biliary cirrhosis (and other causes of hyperbilirubinemia) — Primary biliary cirrhosis, predominantly a disease of females, is characterized by pruritus, obstructive jaundice, elevated levels of alkaline phosphatase, cholesterol and serum IgM. Antimitochondrial antibodies are present in more than 90 per cent of cases.

Iron overload (hemochromatosis) — This rare disorder of iron accumulation may occur as an inherited disease, as a result of repeated transfusions for hematologic problems, in association with cirrhosis and portocaval shunting, or in asssociation with excessive alcohol and iron intake. The skin is bronze or metallic gray due to increased melanin, skin atrophy and iron deposition.

Malignant melanoma — is increasing in prevalence in the United States and is believed to be related to sun exposure. Suggestive clinical features in the primary skin lesion are irregular borders, color variation with mixtures of blue-gray, black, or red and brown, variegation of pigmentation, bleeding, ulceration, a surrounding halo of depigmentation, or satellite nodules. With widespread metastases, precursors of melanin may deposit in the skin resulting in generalized melanosis.

Porphyria — Porphyrins are pigments found principally in hemoglobin and catalase enzymes. There are several forms of porphyria, but skin hyperpigmentation occurs mainly in porphyria cutanea tarda and variegate porphyria. The former type is also characterized by bullae on light exposed or traumatized skin, hypertrichosis and liver disease. The variegate form displays identical skin lesions, acute attacks of abdominal colic and jaundice, psychotic manifestations and a positive Watson-Schwartz test.

Liver disease — Chronic hepatobiliary disorders such as Laennec's cirrhosis frequently cause diffuse brown or dirty tan hyperpigmentation. Occasionally blotchy areas of hypermelanosis may occur. Associated physical findings may include spider angiomas, palmar erythema, gynecomastia, testicular atrophy and Dupuytren's contractures.

Endocrine causes — (see A-C-T-H above)

Drug — Medications including atabrine, busulfan, chloroquine, cytoxan, 5-fluorouracil, bleomycin, nitrogen mustard, psoralen.

Arsenic — a component of some pesticides and Fowler's solution, is also utilized in electroplating and copper processing or smelting. Chronic intoxication may cause neuropathy, as well as central nervous system symptoms of headache, confusion and occasionally convulsions. Dermatologic manifestations include a reticulated brown to gray hyperpigmentation (especially in the trunk, axillae, perineum and pressure sites), palmar and plantar hyperkeratosis with associated yellow papules, and Mees lines (single transverse white bands crossing the nails).

Scleroderma — Skin changes often dominate the clinical appearance, although vital organ involvement determines the course of the disease. Hypermelanosis may be intense and closely resembles Addison's disease, affecting exposed skin and mucous membranes. Morphea, localized sclerotic areas of skin, may be noted or more widespread bound down fibrotic changes may be present. Raynaud's phenomenon with recurrent painful digital ulcers is a frequent early finding.

Sprue (and other malabsorption syndromes such as Whipple's disease) — may cause diffuse hyperpigmentation which is most marked around scars. The buccal mucosa is not affected. Pigmentation may be related to a deficiency of sulfur containing amino acids. There is an association between celiac sprue and dermatitis herpetiformis.

This acronym does not include pellagra and carotinemia.

Chapter 10

The Art of Sensible Living
From the School of Salerno

The formation of the renowned and memorable school of Salerno was one of the most significant events in the history of Medicine. The chronicle of the early centuries of The Middle Ages recorded several illustrious names and important medical events which demonstrate incontestably that even in the most depressing times medical thought continues its advance.

Toward the school of Salerno converged successively all the great currents of medical thought, ancient and contemporary. From the Greek schools of lower Italy and Egypt, from the Monks of Western Europe, from the Jews, Arabs, and Orientals, from the peoples of Northern Europe came an assembly of influences which were absorbed and assimilated in an outstanding secular medical activity. The result was an example of a characteristic Latin trait: that of choosing the liveliest jet of each fountain, the soundest germ of every idea, the unspoiled memory of even the apparently dead past, and giving a practical and lucid turn to every activity. The pleasing bay of Salerno, regarded as an ideal place for sojourn by the Roman physicians, was in that part of Italy where the contacts between races and civilizations were always the liveliest, and where commerce and contact with people from distant lands was the order of the day; here arose the Civitas Hippocratica, the seat of the school of Salerno, a name which retained its fame throughout several centuries.

The school is first spoken of at the beginning of the ninth century, reached its greatest splendor in the twelfth century and preserved its fame to the end of the fourteenth. Throughout its history a distinct tendency toward lay medicine was evident in the character of the instruction to young physicians.

Three periods mark the history of the school. In the first, its

155

widespread reputation attracted patients from distant parts to a hospital founded by the Benedictines toward the end of the seventh century. Information about the early masters is vague, but legend has it that the school was founded by four physicians, a Greek, a Latin, a Jew, and a Saracen. The old Salernitan chronicles tell about a Master Helinus, who read Hebrew lessons to the Jews, a Master Pontus who gave instructions to the Greeks, a Master Adela, an Arab who taught in the Arabian tongue, and a Master Salernus who taught in Latin. Ten physicians comprised the Collegium Hippocraticum, attracting young students of many countries to their lectures. Medical writings of the time, mostly manuals for the students, were almost exclusively summaries or fragments of the old Greek or Latin texts, in which therapy, largely medicinal, without any allusions to magic or astronomy, had the greatest importance.

The best known Salernitan physician of this time was Gariopontus, whose name is connected with an encyclopedic work, *Passionarius,* which had an enviable reputation in the eleventh century as well as later. Although this work is a compilation made from the Latin writings of Galen, Theodorus Priscianus, Alexander of Tralles, and Paul of Aequia, it is of special value because it contains the basis of modern medical terminology. The use of words borrowed from the common tongue shows us that the instruction was intended for the students as well as for the laity. This work gives us a clear picture of the most quoted authors of the period and shows that the dominant force in the teaching at Salerno during this period was the Greco-Latin tradition without Arabian influence.

To the same period belongs another famous physician, Pietro Clerico, or Petroncellus, whose *Practica* prescribes frequent cold baths for a number of diseases. A personality of the first period who has aroused a lively interest among medical historians for a long time is the female physician, Trotula. The book that bears her name, *De Passionibus Mulierum,* reveals considerable practical experience; especially worthy of attention are the rules about the choice of a wet nurse, who should be neither too far from nor too near her last childbirth; a special diet is prescribed, with abstinence from highly salted foods or an excess of pepper and severe prohibition of garlic and onion.

Among the other writings of the period is the celebrated *Antidotarium,* the foundation stone of early Salernitan medicine. A kind of formulary, made up from the daily practices of the hospitals, it was regarded as a canonical book of standards to be followed by the Salernitan physicians in regard to prescriptions for the patients, similar to the formularies that some hospitals of today draw up for the use of their housestaff.

The Golden Period of the School of Salerno — Arabian Winds

The second period of the school of Salerno — That of its greatest splendor — is characterized by the influence of Arabian medicine, which reached it about the end of the eleventh century. The Arabian influence was mostly, though not entirely, due to Constantinus Africanus. From his earliest youth Constantine devoted himself to the study of medicine. His wide knowledge of Oriental languages and his passion for literary studies took him to Salerno where he soon became one of the most esteemed physicians and famed professors of that school. He remained there several years, then became a Benedictine Monk of the Monastery of Montecassino, devoting the rest of his life to intense study until his death in 1087. During his tenure Constantine translated the ancient Oriental texts with more facility than exactness, rewriting everything that came to his hand without distinguishing the rare and precious from mere accumulations of fantasy and extravagence.

Like the Greeks, the doctors of Salerno saw that patients were human, that disease was a natural phenomenon and that common-sense therapies might cure it. The doctor was now called "physicus," or physician, rather than "medicus." The change in terminology emphasized his integration with natural science above and beyond mere medical skill.

Salerno was not a diplomia mill. Roger II and Frederick II of Sicily issued decrees which bound the students to three years work in the humanities, five years specialized training and a final stringent examination before the faculty and the Royal Commissioner. The lucky candidate received a ring, a laurel wreath, a book, and the kiss of peace. Then, after a year's work with an attested physician, the graduate could hang out his own shingle.

To uphold this newly won status the young doctor was required, first, to avoid trouble with the church by seeing that his patient confessed. Next, he needed to win the patient's confidence. A Salernitan tract tells how this was to be achieved: "when the doctor enters the dwelling of his patient, he should greet with kindly, modest demeanor those who are present, and then seating himself near the sick man, accept the drink which is offered him and praise in a few words the beauty of the neighborhood, the situation of the house, and the generosity of the family . . ."

The literary fame of the Salerno school is not due to treatises full of philosophic disquisitions or repetitions of scholastic discussions, but above all to that famous poem, *'Flos Medicinae,* or *Regimen Sanitatis Salernitanum.*

This poem, which includes within itself all the essential didactic characteristics of the school of Salerno, was committed to memory by thousands of physicians, for whom each of these verses had the quality of Holy Writ. It does not, to be sure, constitute a text of medical treatment that conforms to our present ideas of science; but the seductive quality of the verse had the virtue of spreading these useful, simple, and true maxims throughout the entire civilized world, popularizing with good common sense, a sane criticism which bespeaks a Hippocratic quality that is the greatest glory of the school.

Not only were the young doctors of Salerno armed with the verses of *Regimen Sanitatis Salernitanum* but so were the young doctors of other lands. The faculty's surprise best seller quickly spread across Europe. As time went on doctors added new verses to the original 362 and rival schools came out with imitative texts. With the invention of printing, cheap popular versions appeared. By 1852, the book had run to almost 300 editions in many languages, and its verses had grown to 3500.

We quote from this valuable book some of its best known and most popular verses, according to the 1553 editions of Arnold of Villanova's version.

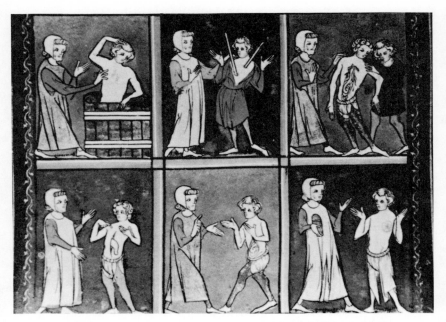

The cover from an early edition of the famed book from the School of Salerno.

The Salerne Schoole doth by
these lines impart
All health to Englands King,
and doth aduise
From care his head to keepe,
from wrath his heart,
Drinke not much wine, sup
light, and soone arise,
When meate is gone, long sit-
ting breedeth smart:
And after-noone still waking
keepe your eyes.
When mou'd you find your
selfe to Natures Needs,
Forbeare them not, for that
much danger breeds,
Use three Physicians still; first
Doctor Quiet,

Next Doctor Merry-man, and
    Doctor Dyet.

Rise early in the morne, and
    straight remember,
With water cold to wash your
    hands and eyes.
In gentle fashion retching
    euery member,
And to refresh your braine
    when as you rise,
In heat, in cold, in July and De-
    cember.
Both comb your head, and rub
    your teeth likewise:
If bled you haue, keep coole, if
    bath'd, keepe warme:
If din'd, to stand or walke will
    do no harme.
But if you still herein exceed to
    farre,
It hurts your health, it cannot
    be with stood:
Long sleepe at after-noones by
    stirring fumes,
Breeds Slouth, and Agues, Ak-
    ing heads and Rheumes:

To keepe good dyet, you
    should neuer feed
Untill you finde your stomacke
    cleane and void
Of former eaten meate, for
    they do breed
Repletion, and will cause you
    soone be cloid,
None other rule but appetite
    should need,

When from your mouth a
    moysture cleare doth
    void.

Egges newly laid, are nutritiue
    to eate,
And rosted Reare are easie to
    digest.
Fresh Gascoigne wine is good
    to drinke with meat,
Broth strengthens nature
    aboue all the rest.

Though all ill sauours do not
    breed infection,
Yet sure infection commeth
    most by smelling,
Some men there are that thinke
    a little nap breeds no ill
    bloud:
In Autumne ware you eate not
    too much fruite:
With Winters cold full meates
    do fittest suite.

If in your drinke you mingle
    Rew with Sage,
All poyson is expeld by power
    of those,
And if you would withall Lusts
    heat asswage,
Adde to them two the gentle
    flowre of Rose:
Would not be sea-sicke when
    seas do rage,
Sage-water drinke with wine
    before he goes.
Of washing of your hands
    much good doth rise,

Tis wholesome, cleanely, and
    relieues your eyes.

Porke without wine is not so
    good to eate,
As Sheepe with wine, it medi-
    cine is and meate,
Tho Intrailes of a beast be not
    the best,
Yet are some intrailes better
    than the rest.

'Tis good a Goat or Camels
    milke to drinke,
Cowes-milke and Sheepes doe
    well, but yet an Asses
Is best of all, and all the others
    passes.

To close your stomack well,
    this order sutes,
In Spring your dinner must not
    much exceed,
In Summers heate but little
    meate shall need:

Cheese after flesh, Nuts after
    fish or fruits,
Yet some haue said, (beleeue
    them as you will)
One Nut doth good, two hurt,
    the third doth kill.

But who can write thy worth (O
    soueraigne Sage!).
Some aske how man can die,
    where thou dost grow,
Oh that there were a medicine
    curing age,
Death comes at last, though

death comes ne're so
slow:
Sage strengths the sinewes,
seuere heat doth swage,
The Palsy helpes, and rids of
mickle woe.

These are the things that breed
it [our hearing] most of-
fence,
To sleepe on stomacke full and
drinking hard,
Blowes, fals, and noyse, and
fasting violence,
Great heate and sodaine cool-
ing afterwards;
All these, as is by sundry
proofes appearing,
Breed tingling in our eares, and
hurt our hearing:

Now shall you see what hurt-
full is for sight:
Wine, women, Bathes, by art
to nature wrought,
Leekes, Onyons, Garlicke,
Mustard seed, fire and
light,
Smoake, bruises, dust, Pepper
to powder brought,
Beanes, Lentiles, strains,
Wind, Tears, & Phoebus
bright,
And all sharpe things our eye-
sight do molest:
Yet watching hurts them more
then all the rest.

Make your incision large and

not to deepe
That bloud have speedy issue
    with the fume
So that from sinewes you all
    hurt do keepe
Nor may you (as I tougt before)
    presume
In six houres at all to sleepe
Lest some slight bruise in sleep
    cause an apostume.

The spring is moist, of temper
    good and warme,
Then best it is to bathe, to
    sweate, and purge,
Then may one ope a veine in
    either arme,
If boyling bloud or feare of
    agues vrge:
Then Venus recreation doth no
    harme,
Yet may too much thereof
    turne to a scourge.
In Summers heat (when choller
    hath dominion)
Coole meates and moist are
    best in some opinion:
The Fall is like the Spring, but
    endeth colder,
With wines and Spice the Win-
    ter may be bolder.

Later versions of the poem as well as new additions contained specific herbal remedies for gout, phlegm or ague and relatively sound advice about diet, sleep, sex, drink and diversion. These were written in an Anglicized form and included a number of don'ts: don't read in bed, don't drink too much, don't love too much, and don't strain at stool too much. Others are listed below:

If thou to health and vigor wouldst attain
Shun weighty cares — all anger deem profane
From heavy suppers and much wine abstain.

Use three physicians still — first Dr. Diet
Next Dr. Merryman, third Dr. Quiet.

Great suppers will the stomach's peace impair
Wouldst lightly rest — curtail thine evening fare.

Shun idle slumber nor delay
The urgent calls of nature to obey.

Nor trivial count is after pompous fare
To rise from table and to take the air.

Let doctors call in clothing fine arrayed
With sparkling jewels on their hands displayed
For when well dressed and looking over nice
They may presume to charge a higher price.

But as all practice shows, no doctor can
Make life anew, though he may stretch its span.

"If in your teeth you hap to be tormented
Burn Frankincense (a gum not evil scented)
And in a tunnel to the tooth that's hollow,
Convey the smoke thereof, and ease shall follow."

Thus the Regimen became a kind of folk epic, a guidebook for the home, containing the medical experience of an entire continent. The Salernitan stamp of simplicity and closeness to daily life insured its popular appeal. The jingles were easy to memorize, they left no doubt about what to do or what to avoid.

In later editions, when the more ponderous scholars fell victim to the seductive charm of the book, some lengthy rhapsodies appeared on climate and disease, the four humors, venesection, and uroscopy. Such verses provided the profession with indispensable precepts, and thousands of physicians committed these to memory. In this way the Regimen finally became the backbone of all practical medical literature up to the 18th century. Salernitan wisdom is heeded even today in the medical folklore of Europe and America.

Chapter 11

Mnemonics:

Neurology

What is sometimes called clinical instinct . . . may be lacking in men of high intellectual ability and present to a marked degree in those who are . . . mentally their inferiors. It seems to be much the same as common sense and closely allied to a sense of humour, which is the same thing as a sense of proportion.

If the natural powers of judgement are to be improved it is only . . . by general mental culture and not by purely scientific training that it can be done . . . I regret the modern tendency to make the scientific studies of the medical student begin at an earlier age . . . and to sacrifice to them much of the old literary and linguistic training. It is . . . not without significance . . . that many of the most distinguished physicians . . . have also been good classical scholars.

Sir Robert Hutchison
The Principles of Diagnosis
British Medical Journal 1928

Peripheral Neuropathy

Peripheral neuropathy is one of the most perplexing problems that can confront the clinician. In as many as half of the patients with peripheral nerve disease, a clear explanation of the reasons for this difficulty is never discovered. Perhaps the mnemonic which follows will aid the examiner in considering the long list of possible causes.

The origin of the word "nerve" can be traced back to the Sanskrit "nauree" which means "a string." The Greek physicians used the derived word for a nerve, tendon or ligament if it took the form of a cord. The term neuron was used by Hippocrates for any white cord-like structure. This overlap, which sometimes created confusion among later anatomists, is still evident in the term, aponeurosis; an expansion of fibrous tissue from a tendon, a broad piece of tissue or, if you'll allow us our poetic license, a BROAD LIGAMENT.

Acrostic for the Causes of Peripheral Neuropathy:
B-R-O-A-D   L-I-G-A-M-E-N-T-S*

B-vitamin deficiency — Included among this class is beriberi, a disease of the heart and peripheral nerves. In most cases, the polyneuropathy affects only the limbs and alcoholism is frequently associated. Niacin deficiency (pellagra) generally produces cerebral manifestations but may cause a peripheral neuropathy indistinguishable from beriberi. The spinal cord, brain, optic nerves and peripheral nerves may all be involved in vitamin B_{12} deficiency. The spinal cord is often affected first and may demonstrate subacute combined degeneration of the cord.

Renal failure — Polyneuropathy is a common complication of chronic renal failure leading to a painless, progressive, symmetrical paralysis of the legs and then of the arms. Occasionally, burning dysesthesias may be present in the lower extremities. Usually the neuropathy evolves over many months, but improvement is afforded by hemodialysis and recovery follows successful renal transplantation.

Oncovin (vincristine) — Paresthesias of the extremeties may occur within a few weeks of the onset of treatment with this chemotherapeutic agent. With continued use a progressive motor-sensory loss ensues. Cranial nerves and the autonomic nervous system are less frequently affected.

Amyloidosis — may occur secondary to prolonged inflammatory disease or in association with familial Mediterranean fever, multiple myeloma, or macroglobulinemia. Sporadic primary amyloidosis, localized amyloidosis and specific genetic forms also exist. In all these forms, pathologic examination may reveal amyloid deposition in blood vessels and intersti-

168

tial tissues of peripheral nerves, and occasionally in the spinal and autonomic ganglia and roots.

Diabetes — Nearly 50 per cent of diabetics either have neuropathic symptoms or exhibit slowed nerve conduction velocities. A distal, symmetric, slowly progressive, primarily sensory polyneuropathy is the most common form. Other clinical syndromes include diabetic ophthalmoplegia, acute mononeuropathy, an asymmetric, motor, multiple neuropathy (mononeuropathy multiplex), and an autonomic neuropathy affecting bowel, bladder, and circulatory reflexes.

Lead (see the ABC's of lead poisoning p. 15) — Chronic exposure to lead may produce a predominantly motor neuropathy characteristically involving the upper extremities. The radial nerves are the most commonly affected, producing wrist drop.

Infectious mononucleosis and **I**nfectious hepatitis — may both be associated with an ascending sensory-motor paralysis of the Landry-Guillain-Barre variety. With mononucleosis, meningoencephalitis and aseptic meningitis have also been described.

Guillain-Barre syndrome — usually follows a mild respiratory or gastrointestinal infection in 1 to 3 weeks time. It may also follow surgical procedures, antirabies inoculation or may accompany Hodgkin's disease. The most prominent manifestation is weakness which usually evolves over several days. In the majority of cases, paralysis ascends from legs to trunk, arms and cranial nerves, peaking in severity within 10 to 14 days. Variants, however, are frequent and the weakness can progress to motor paralysis with death from respiratory failure within a few days.

Arsenic (or alternatively **A**rteritis) — Arsenic induced polyneuropathy is similar to that noted in beriberi. Other metals such as mercury, antimony and thallium may also produce a peripheral neuropathy. In 10 to 20 per cent of patients with polyarteritis nodosa, a symptomatic form of neuropathy develops.

Malignancy — A slowly developing symmetric sensory-motor or pure sensory peripheral neuropathy may accompany carcinomas, multiple myeloma, solitary plasmacytomas, or macroglobulinemia. Improvement may follow removal of the tumor or control of the underlying malignancy.

Ethyl alcohol — Alcoholic polyneuropathy is due to a combination of alcoholic abuse and associated deficiencies of essential B-vitamins. After several months of dietary inadequacy, sensory-motor neuropathy develops first in the distal lower extremities. With time, the proximal leg and upper extremities may be involved, although cranial structures are always spared unless Wernicke's disease coexists.

Nitrofurantoin neuropathy — produces tingling dysesthesias of the feet and hands after high dose administration of the medication for weeks or months. Those patients with renal impairment are particularly prone to this complication, which may progress to a severe sensory-motor neuropathy unless the drug is discontinued.

Trauma — External trauma or a period of prolonged compression of a nerve against underlying bone may result in paralysis and sensory loss in the corresponding region supplied by the nerve. (e.g. Saturday-night palsy).

Sarcoidosis — is a rare cause of asymmetric polyneuropathy. It may be associated with polymyositis and signs of central nervous system involvement. Isolated facial palsy is the most frequent site of peripheral nerve involvement.

This list lacks diphtheritic and porphyric polyneuropathies, leprosy, organic toxins and hereditary neuropathic syndromes.

Another mnemonic for peripheral polyneuropathies which uses a more general approach to the subject is given here:

Mnemonic: D-A-N-G   T-He-R-A-P-I-S-T

Diabetic

Alcoholic

Nutritional

Guillain-Barre

Toxic — lead, arsenic, thalidomide, mercury, organophosphorous compounds, nitrofurantoin, vincristine.

Hereditary disorders — such as 1) Dejerine-Sottas neuropathy, a hypertrophic polyneuropathy in which there are palpably enlarged nerves, 2) Refsum's disease, which is associated with ataxia, retinitis pigmentosa, enlarged nerves, deafness, and elevated serum phytanic acid and 3) Charcot-Marie-Tooth disease, characterized by clubbed feet, and peroneal muscular atrophy.

Recurrent polyneuropathy (chronic progressive, idiopathic) — sometimes responds to steroid administration.

Amyloidosis — slowly progressive, occasionally painful.

Porphyric polyneuropathy — is a symmetric, rapidly progressive form that affects principally the motor nerves of patients with acute intermittent porphyria.

Infectious causes — diphtheria, mononucleosis, hepatitis, leprosy.

Systemic — polyneuropathies associated with systemic diseases such as sarcoidosis, uremia, and collagen vascular disorders.

Tumors

Charcot

Its been about 120 years since Charcot became the chief physician for the 4,000 bed Salpetriere, a house of refuge for aged women. His name has been included in many eponymic syndromes, symptoms and signs. Some of his more notable observations are remembered with respect here.

Mnemonic: CH-AR-CO-T-'S   GR-E-AT*

CH — Cerebral Hemorrhage — Charcot's artery of cerebral hemorrhage is the early name for the lenticulostriate branch of the middle cerebral artery.

AR — Arthritis — Charcot's joint is a late manifestation of neuropathies, especially tabes dorsalis or syringomyelia. The affected joint, usually an ankle or knee, is characterized by painless enlargement and deformity, with hypermobility and absence of inflammation.

CO — Cough — Charcot-Leyden crystals are found wherever eosinophils are undergoing fragmentation; such as in the sputum of asthmatics.

T — Temperature — Charcot's intermittent fever. In some instances, gallstones lodged in the common bile duct may be painless and produce only recurrent fever and chills.

S — Sclerosis — Charcot's disease is the early name for disseminated sclerosis of the nervous system; multiple sclerosis.

GR — Graves disease — Charcot-Vigouroux sign is a diminished electrical resistance noted in the skin of patients with hyperthyroidism.

E — Ejaculate — Charcot-Neumman crystals, composed of spermine phosphate, were first described by Charcot.

AT — Atherosclerosis — Charcot's sign is intermittent limping and claudication noted in those persons affected by atherosclerosis of the arteries supplying the lower extremities.

Diffuse Hyperreflexia

Interruption of the corticospinal tract causes disinhibition of spinal motor mechanisms and leads to enhanced muscle stretch reflexes and, at times, associated spasticity.

The S's of Diffuse Hyperreflexia:*

Sclerosis (Multiple sclerosis and amyotrophic lateral sclerosis): — Hyperreflexia tends to be a late sign of multiple sclerosis. Early signs vary from patient to patient and include weakness and/or numbness in one or more limbs, retrobulbar neuritis, unsteadiness of gait or brainstem symptoms. The classic triad of amyotrophic lateral sclerosis includes atrophic weakness of the hands and forearms, slight spasticity of the legs, and generalized hyperreflexia, all in the absence of sensory symptoms.

Spinal cord compression — (See the symptoms and signs of spinal cord compression S-H-A-R-P W-A-L-L p. 143). After a period of areflexia, complete severance of the spinal cord is followed, in several weeks, by hyperreflexia. Less severe compression of the spinal cord is manifested by hyperreflexia early on in the development of various disorders such as . . .

Spondylosis of the cervical spine.

Spastic paraplegia (familial forms) — This group consists of several hereditary disorders and includes Werdnig-Hoffman disease, Wohlfart-Kugelberg-Welunder syndrome, familial forms of ALS, Fazio-Londe syndrome, Ferguson-Critchley syndrome, and syndromes of spastic paraplegia associated with optic and retinal degenerations.

Sagittal intracranial masses may present as hyperreflexia.

Strokes — Multiple strokes may lead to diffuse hyperreflexia by causing widespread derangement of upper motor neurons.

Serebral palsy — (cerebral palsy — please pardon the cepelling) is the designation for a wide variety of neurologic disorders in which major motor function disturbances have been present since infancy. Proper understanding of these diseases requires understanding of the etiologic and developmental factors involved in each individual case.

Scirrhosis (Once again, sorry about the spelling) — Hepatic encephalopathy is a clinical picture consisting of mental confusion, stupor or coma, asterixis (liver-flap), fairly specific EEG findings, pathological reflexes and hyperreflexia. Uremic encephalopathy may present a similar picture.

Myopathies

A sudden paralysis of skeletal muscles in one region of the body is usually due to a vascular problem in the central nervous system. Acute paralysis developing over several days to 1 or 2 weeks is usually due to one of the polyneuropathies such as Guillain-Barre. The course of primary muscle disorders, in contrast is subacute, covering the time span of several weeks.

An Epi-acronym for Remembering the Major Myopathies:*

Polly's — Perilous — Thighs
Could — Crush — Al's
Muscular — Mastadon

Polly's — Polymyositis — Polymyositis is a disease affecting the proximal limb and trunk muscles. The muscles, which are usually not tender, reveal widespread destruction of muscle fibers and inflammatory infiltrate on biopsy. In dermatomyositis, skin changes are also present and take the form of localized or diffuse erythema, maculopapular eruptions, scaling eczematoid dermatitis or the characteristic heliotrope rash.

Perilous — Periodic paralysis — This is generally a hereditary disease which has its onset in late childhood or adolescence. The typical attack occurs during sleep following a day of strenuous exercise and is associated with a reduction in the serum potassium level. Generally, the limbs are affected more than the trunk, especially the proximal muscles of the lower extremities. Pathologically, the most striking finding is vacuolization of the sarcoplasm.

Thighs — Thyroid — Several myopathic disorders have been associated with altered thyroid function. These include: 1) chronic thyrotoxic myopathy characterized by progressive weakness and atrophy of muscles, especially those of the pelvic girdle and thighs, 2) thyrotoxic periodic paralysis which resembles the familial form described above, 3) myasthenia gravis which may accompany diffuse toxic goiter and, 4) muscle hypertrophy and slow muscle contraction associated with hypothyroidism.

Could — Corticosteroid — In most patients suffering from steroid myopathy the corticosteroid dose has been high and sustained over months to years. The proximal muscles are most severely affected and biopsies disclose atrophic fibers and the absence of inflammatory cells. A similar myopathy occurs commonly in patients with . . .

Crush — Cushing's syndrome — The mechanism of the muscle disease in either corticosteroid-induced or Cushing's myopathy is unknown.

Al's — Alcohol — Alcoholic myopathy may take the form of a proximal weakness developing over days to weeks during a long drinking bout. This form is associated with hypokalemia and biopsy findings of fiber necrosis and vacuolization. Another syndrome, in which painful edema of the limb and trunk musculature is associated with hyperkalemia and renal damage, may occur acutely during a severe drinking bout.

Muscular — Muscular dystrophies — This category of diseases includes different varieties of inherited disorders. The Duchenne type begins in infancy and childhood, is severe and is usually sex linked. Classically, the calves (and sometimes the quadriceps and deltoids) show pseudohypertrophy early in the disease. Other less common forms of muscular dystrophy include fascioscapulohumeral dystrophy, limb-girdle dystrophy of Erb, a distal type of dystrophy, myotonic dystrophy, and an ophthalmoplegic or oculopharyngeal dystrophy.

Mastadon — Myasthenia — Myasthenia gravis is a disorder characterized by fluctuating weakness of voluntary muscles, especially ocular, masticatory, facial, deglutitional and lingual muscles. Repeated activity of the affected muscle groups leads to exhaustion of their contractility and rest partially restores strength. Thymic tumors and/or hyperplasia of the gland are frequently associated with the disease. Thymectomy induces remission in as many as 50 per cent of patients.

Aphasia

Better to remain silent and be thought a fool than to speak out and remove all doubt.

— Abraham Lincoln

Look wise, say nothing and grunt.

— William Osler

It is important to differentiate between aphasia, in which the affected individual uses language incorrectly or comprehends it imperfectly, and dysarthria, in which the patient articulates poorly but language content, form and usage are normal.

The following stanzas serve as reminders to the classification of the five main kinds of aphasia.*

Broken hearts
  are **not fully reparable**
  and that's **understandable.**

In Broca's aphasia:
  The patient is
  not fluent, repeats
  well and
  understands well.

Working parts
  are made **irreparable**
  by **foolish misunderstanding.**

In Wernicke's aphasia:
  The patient
  repeats poorly, is
  fluent and can't understand.

Worldly ambition is
  neither foolish nor irreparable
  but is totally **incomprehensi-
  ble.**

In Global aphasia:
  The patient
  is not fluent, can't
  repeat and
  can't comprehend.

Conduct your life
  **flawlessly, compromise
  without a word**
  and **avoid reprimanding.**

In Conductive aphasia:
  The patient
  is fluent, comprehends
  well, displays anomia,
  and repeats poorly.

Though **anonymous**
  you **remain**
with **no name** at all
  you will be **full** of
    understanding.

In Anomic aphasia:
  The patient repeats well,
  has difficulty naming
  objects, is fluent and
  understands.

Non-dominant Cerebral Hemispheric Findings

The functional dominance of one cerebral hemisphere is important in the development of language function. Left dominance is present in greater than 95 per cent of the general population and is associated with greater facility in the use of the right hand, foot, and eye. Handedness, in fact, develops simultaneously with language. However, studies of aphasia in left handed individuals have revealed that 75 per cent of them had left cerebral hemispheric lesions. In the rare cases of aphasia due to right cerebral lesions, the patient is virtually always left-handed. With these thoughts in mind, the clinician must remember to test most carefully for non-dominant hemispheric findings when confronted with a patient with a left hemiplegia.

Mnemonic for Non-Dominant Hemispheric Findings:
D-E-N-I-A-L-S*

Anton is credited with first observing that a patient with a dense left hemiplegia may be indifferent to or unaware of his or her mental and physical deficiencies. The patient may display:

Dressing apraxia — The individual ignores one side of the body in proper dressing. The patient may put the left shoe on the right foot or vice versa.

Extinction phenomena — On simultaneous sensory stimulation of corresponding body parts (e.g. touching the backs of both hands), the patient recognizes the stimulation on the intact side only. On separately testing the areas the individual can recognize the stimuli normally.

Neglectfulness — The patient may ignore the left side of the body in grooming and act as if nothing is the matter. If asked to move the paralyzed limb the person may lift the intact one. If confronted with this inconsistency, he may deny it or offer an excuse such as — "my shoulder hurts." Some patients may even deny that the affected extremity belongs to them.

Impersistence of task — When asked to do a simple task such as sticking one's tongue out, the individual may be unable or unwilling to maintain this simple posture.

Apraxia of construction — The patient may be unable to copy simple diagrams such as a cube or clock.

Left-right confusion — Ask the patient to raise his left hand or touch his left ear with his right hand in order to test for this.

Spatial disorientation — The individual may be unable to find the way back to his or her room after being led down the hall.

Vertigo and Disequilibrium

A careful history is essential in distinguishing dizziness from true vertigo. The examiner must be persistent in clearly defining the patient's sensations. All but the mildest varieties of true vertigo are associated with some degree of nausea, vomiting, pallor or sweating. After establishing that the patient is experiencing vertigo, it becomes useful to determine if the vertigo has its origin in peripheral structures (the ear and associated structures) or in the central nervous system. A chart containing distinguishing characteristics of these two forms of vertigo is provided in the appendix (p. 213).

In the mnemonic below, the word aplomb, used to mean assurance or poise, originates from the French term meaning "according to the plumb bob"; in other words, being perpendicular, upright or vertical. In ballet "aplomb" refers to the equilibrium required to maintain stability in a particular pose.

Mnemonic for Causes of Vertigo and Disequilibrium:
A-B-S-E-N-T   A-P-L-O-M-B*

Arrythmias — Sudden onset and cessation of palpitation, dyspnea, or presyncope may suggest this diagnosis. A baseline ECG, exercise ECG, and holter monitor are useful screening and diagnostic tools in determining whether arrythmias are causing disequilibrium.

Blood pressure elevation or depression — Hypotension may occur due to postural changes or may be associated with activity in patients with aortic valve stenosis and other causes of restricted systemic cardiac output. Severe hypertension may also occasionally produce symptoms of vertigo or disequilibrium.

Subclavian steal — is an uncommon disorder due to atherosclerotic narrowing of the subclavian artery proximal to the origin of the vertebral artery. Exercise of the arm causes reversal of blood flow in the vertebral artery and associated symptoms of vertigo, diplopia, dysarthria and, occasionally, syncope.

Epilepsy — Temporal lobe epilepsy is characterized by a varied combination of signs including brief absence or staring spells, automatisms, such as facial grimacing and lip smacking, rage reactions and deja vu or jamais vu-like sensations. Vertigo may occur as an aura in this form of seizure or in grand mal or psychomotor seizures. Occasionally, vertigo is the sole manifestation of the seizure. One should suspect epilepsy, especially in the situation when loss of consciousness occurs during a vertiginous episode.

Neuronitis (vestibular neuronitis) — A recent history of bacterial or viral illness followed by the acute onset of severe vertigo with nausea and vomiting should suggest this diagnosis. In contrast to Meniere's disease, tinnitus and deafness are absent and the episode endures for several days rather than minutes or hours.

Trauma — Concussion of the inner ear, basilar fracture involving the petrous temporal bone or cervical injury such as whiplash may all produce vertigo. In whiplash injury, the vertigo may be due to involvement of the cervical sensory afferent fibers and may be triggered when the individual turns his head toward the side of the injury.

Acoustic neuromas — originate in the internal auditory canal and symptoms develop as the tumor compresses the eighth cranial nerve. The clinician may elicit a history of tinnitus and unilateral hearing loss. Vertigo occurs in approximately one third of patients. Other neurologic symptoms such as facial weakness and loss of the corneal reflex develop as the tumor spreads beyond the internal auditory canal.

Paroxysmal positional vertigo — Vertigo initiated by specific head positions points to this diagnosis. The vertigo typically begins after a latent period of 2-20 seconds, lasts for 20-30 seconds and is not accompanied by hearing difficulties.

Labyrinthitis — is another vestibular disorder with a similar constellation of symptoms as that noted in vestibular neuronitis. However, tinnitus and hearing loss will also be present.

Ototoxins — Substances include alcohol, aminoglycoside antibiotics, phenytoin, barbiturates, birth control pills, caffeine, ethacrynic acid, furosemide, quinidine, salicylates, sedative hypnotics, minocycline, and tobacco.

Meniere's disease — presents with the symptom triad of episodic vertigo, fluctuating hearing loss and tinnitus. The attacks of vertigo usually last between 30 minutes to 3 hours and are dramatic, accompanied by nausea and vomiting. The pathogenesis of the disorder is an increase in the volume of endolymph which, in turn, causes mechanical and neurosensory dysfunction of the cochlear and vestibular end organs.

Basilar migraine or ischemia — Basilar migraine may produce vertigo followed by a throbbing occipital headache. The patient often reports an aura composed of scintillating scotomata and homonymous hemianopsia. In older individuals one of the most common causes of vertigo is vertebral basilar artery insufficiency. T.I.A.'s in this distribution usually produce multiple symptoms. Many of these symptoms start with the letter 'D'; dizziness or disequilibrium, dysarthria, dysphagia, diplopia, demi(hemi)paresis, demianesthesia, double homonymous hemianopsia.

This list excludes several causes of vertigo; lateral medullary syndrome (Wallenberg's syndrome), cerebellar hemorrhage or infarction and multiple sclerosis.

Signs of Cerebellar Disease

The most prominent manifestations of cerebellar disease are those related to incoordination of voluntary motion. The dyssynergy of cerebellar disorders can often be demonstrated by having the patient attempt simple hand movements such as pronating and supinating the hands in rapid succession, finger-to-nose testing, or rhythmic clapping of the hands.

Acronym for the Signs of Cerebellar Disease:
H-A-N-D-S*

Hypotonia — is a fundamental sign of cerebellar disorders but is more apparent with acute than with chronic lesions. There may be undue flabbiness of the muscles ipsilateral to the cerebellar lesion. The Stewart-Holmes rebound sign may be present. In this test, the patient flexes his arm against resistance. In cerebellar disease, sudden release of the arm may cause rebound in several cycles of flexion and extension or the patient may actually be unable to prevent striking himself. Defective contraction of the quadriceps and hamstring muscles cause a pendulous patellar reflex, another manifestation of hypotonia.

Asynergy — Dyssynergy, dysmetria and dysdiadokinesis are related disturbances in the rate, range and force of movement. The velocity and initiation of movement are only slightly affected in cerebellar disorders, but the fluidity of motion is deranged. These abnormalities are most prominent as the patient's finger or toe approaches a target. During the limb's excursion toward its objective, jerky movements or past-pointing are noted; motions composed of a series of imprecise voluntary movements, each trying to correct its predecessor.

Nystagmus — Decomposition of movements may also be noted in ocular motion in individuals with cerebellar disease. Ocular oscillations are seen as the eyes approach and then overshoot their target. Although this may not represent true nystagmus, large lesions of the cerebellar cortex which involve the fastigiovestibular fibers do produce nystagmus unrelated to ocular past-pointing.

Dysarthria — Scanning speech is characterized by a slow, broken-up series of improperly emphasized syllables punctuated with involuntary interruptions (explosive speech).

<u>S</u>tation and gait difficulties — The features of the cerebellar gait include unsteadiness with reeling toward the affected side of the body, irregularity of steps and separation of the legs (broad-based gait). The ataxia is not ameliorated by visual orientation, as in the disordered proprioception of posterior column disease, in which Romberg's sign is positive. When mild, the gait abnormality is best demonstrated by having the patient walk heel to toe in a line. Tested in this manner, the patient will lose his balance and will find it necessary to extend his foot sideways to avoid falling.

Dementia

"Body and mind, like man and wife, do not always agree to die together."

— C.C. Colton

Dementia comes from the Latin word "dementio," meaning "out of one's mind." Delirium has a similar definition but usually signifies a more temporary disorder of the mental faculties and has

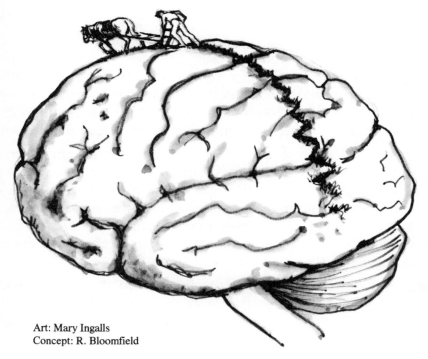

Art: Mary Ingalls
Concept: R. Bloomfield

the connotation of associated violent emotional displays. The term "delirium" has been traced back to the Latin "de," meaning from and "lira" meaning furrow; to go out of the furrow while plowing; to wander from the decidedly normal course.

Acrostic for Major Causes of Dementia:
T-I-L-L   U-P   F-A-S-T   W-I-T-H   P-L-O-W-S*

Tumor — Primary or metastatic brain tumors may produce general cerebral symptoms such as headache, vomiting, stupor or psychic changes. Primary tumors likely in causing dementia include the highly malignant glioblastoma multiforme, the slower growing astrocytoma, and the rarer oligodendrocytoma and ependymoma. Meningiomas produce symptoms by compression of neighboring brain tissue. The major causes of metastatic central nervous system disease are cancers of the lung, breast, colon and kidney.

Intoxication — such as bromidism or chronic barbiturate intoxication.

Lipid storage disease — Lipidoses of the nervous system are characterized by abnormal accumulations of lipids in the brain and other organs. Many varieties exist, including Tay-Sachs disease of infants and the related juvenile and adult forms of this syndrome: Neimann-Pick disease, Hunter-Hurler syndrome, and Gaucher's disease.

Leukodystrophies — The principal pathologic features of these disorders is diffuse disintegration of myelin in the nervous system. This group includes Schilder's disease, metachromatic leukodystrophy, Krabbe's leukodystrophy, late-life leukodystrophy, and Pelizaeus-Merzbacher disease.

Uremia — Uremic encephalopathy may take many forms. Confusion, apathy, and irritability are common early signs. Visual hallucinations may occasionally occur as an isolated manifestation. A twitch-convulsive syndrome in which tremors, fasciculations myoclonus or convulsions may ensue, has also been described. Dialysis dementia occasionally complicates chronic hemodialysis and is associated with seizures and myoclonus.

Pick's disease — is a progressive disorder featuring circumscribed cerebral atrophy. It is indistinguishable from the much more common diffuse atrophy of Alzheimer's disease.

Fahn's disease — is a familial calcification of vessels in the basal ganglia and is manifested by choreoathetosis and dementia which have their onset in adolescence or early adult life. Hypoparathyroidism may produce similar pathologic and clinical findings.

Alzheimer's disease — is the most frequent cause of dementia. Its onset is often insidious and its course is one of progressive deterioration of the mental faculties, especially the memory. Pathologically the brain tissue reveals diffuse atrophy, widespread loss of nerve cells, senile plaques and neurofibrillary tangles.

Strokes — Multiple ischemic insults to the brain lead to impairment of cortical functions. It is doubtful that diffuse arteriosclerotic disease in the absence of strokes produces dementia.

Trauma — such as cerebral contusion, midbrain hemorrhage or chronic subdural hematomas can cause dementia. Posttraumatic hydrocephalus may complicate any severe head injury.

Wernicke-Korsakoff syndrome — occurs most commonly in the nutritionally deficient alcoholic. This combined syndrome displays ataxia of gait, nystagmus, abducens and conjugate gaze difficulties and a unique intellectual impairment, especially with regard to short-term memory and immediate recall. Confabulation is a feature of most cases.

Infection — Chronic infections such as neurosyphilis, cryptococcus, tuberculosis, and viral infections such as herpes simplex encephalalitis, kuru (Creutzfeldt-Jakob disease) and subacute sclerosing panencephalitis.

Thyroid disease — Psychomotor retardation, slow speech, apathy and memory disturbances are common in hypothyroidism.

Huntington's chorea — is a dominantly inherited disorder which features emotional lability, choreoathetosis, and dementia. Atrophy of the heads of the caudate nuclei and putamen are the characteristic pathological findings. The central nervous system degenerates progressively leading to death, on an average, 15 years after onset.

Parkinson's disease (paralysis agitans) — In long standing disease and in patients on long term L-dopa therapy, dementia may supervene. Extrapyramidal symptoms and signs are invariably present; e.g. a resting tremor (most pronounced in the hands with a frequency of 4-8 per second), a festinating gait, and hypokinesia.

Liver failure — Hepatic encephalopathy occurs when substantial portacaval shunting allows ammonium and other amines to enter the systemic circulation. Mental confusion, drowsiness, stupor, and, finally, coma may evolve over a period of days to weeks unless steps are taken to reverse exascerbating factors (e.g. dehydration, infection or gastrointestinal bleeding).

Occult hydrocephalus (normal pressure hydrocephalus) — refers to a reversible syndrome in which ventricular enlargement occurs without cortical atrophy. It is due to inadequate reabsorption of cerebrospinal fluid and presents clinically with gait disturbances, incontinence and dementia.

Wilson's disease (hepatolenticular degeneration) — is an autosomal recessive inherited disorder in which liver, kidney, brain and cornea are damaged by excessive copper. The most frequent mode of presentation is that of progressive hepatic insufficiency. The most unique finding is the Kayser-Fleischer ring of pigment seen at the periphery of the cornea.

Sclerosis (multiple sclerosis) — Longstanding multiple sclerosis with a history of remissions may eventually cause dementia. Optic atrophy, brain stem signs, and spinal cord signs will usually also be present.

Coma

In their treatise on *The Diagnosis of Stupor and Coma,* Plum and Posner reviewed a group of 386 patients admitted to the hospital with the diagnosis of "coma of unknown etiology." Approximately 68 per cent of their cases were due to metabolic or diffuse cerebral processes, including exogenous toxins, endogenous toxins, brain anoxia, infections and postictal states. Supratentorial mass lesions such as subdural or intracerebral hematomas, and brain tumors were causative in 18 per cent of patients. About 13 per cent were due to subtentorial lesions including brain stem infarcts or hemorrhage and cerebellar hemorrhage. A few cases of coma were secondary to psychiatric disorders.

Two well-known acronyms for recalling numerous causes of coma are given below;

Mnemonic #1:
A-E-I-O-U   T-I-P-S

A — Alcoholism — e.g. intoxication, withdrawal, Wernicke's encephalopathy, associated head trauma, hypoglycemia, hypothermia, delirium tremens.

E — Encephalopathy — e.g. hyperviscosity syndromes, thrombotic thrombocytopenic purpura, normal pressure hydrocephalus, status epilepticus and postictal states, mass lesions, electrolyte abnormalities (hyponatremia, hypercalcemia), hypoxia, hypercapnia, severe hypertension.

I — Insulin excess or deficiency — diabetic ketoacidosis, nonketotic hyperosmolar coma, hypoglycemia.

O — Opiates — narcotics and other exogenous toxins

U — Uremia and other metabolic abnormalities or endogenous toxins (e.g. Addison's disease, myxedema, lactic acidosis, hepatic encephalopathy, porphyria).

T — Trauma — e.g. cerebral contusions, subdural or epidural hematomas, subarachnoid hemorrhage, concussion.

I — Infection — e.g. viral encephalitis, meningitis, brain abscess, pneumonia (may precipitate delirium or coma in the elderly).

P — Psychiatric — e.g. hysteric reaction, schizophrenic reaction.

S — Syncope — cardiovascular causes such as Stokes-Adams attacks, syncope associated with aortic stenosis, or any cause of reduced cardiac output.

Mnemonic #2

I S-P-O-U-T   A   V-E-I-N

Insulin

Shock

Psychogenic

Opiates and other drugs

Uremia and other metabolic derangements

Trauma

Alcohol

Vascular accidents

Encephalopathies

Infection

Neoplasms

In closing this chapter, we'd like to leave our readers with a simple neurological pearl: it is easier for a patient with Parkinson's disease to bicycle than to walk.

Chapter 12
Mnemonics:

Miscellaneous

Some people don't have enough brains to become doctors; others have too much.

M.A. Perlstein

And unless you need them for preserving specimens of the local flora or maintaining the creases upon your Sunday trousers, you should never never never pack technical books into a holiday trunk. It is to put poison, or at any rate, water, into the wine that you are to pour out before the gods of mountains and moor and loch.

Peter Harding M.D.
The Corner of Harley St.

Now I do protest in the name of common sense, against all such proceedings as this. It is very fine to insist that the eye cannot be understood without a knowledge of optics, nor the circulation without mechanics . . . It is a truth and it is a truth also that the whole circle of science is required to comprehend a single particle of matter; but the most solemn truth of all is that the life of man is three score years and ten.

Latham.

Prolactin Excess

Prolactin levels may be elevated in both men and women and yet cause no recognizable symptoms. In fact, only one out of six women with high prolactin secretion will demonstrate the clinical nonpuerperal hallmarks of this abnormality; galactorrhea and amenorrhea. In affected males, infertility and impotence are the usual manifestations. On the other hand, galactorrhea and amenorrhea can be present with normal serum prolactin levels.

Acronym for Causes of Increased Serum Prolactin:
H-I-G-H   P-R-O-L-A-C-T-I-N*

Hypertensive medications (reserpine, alpha-methyldopa) — In addition to the hypothalamic inhibition of prolactin secretion (mediated by prolactin inhibitory factor; P.I.H.), dopamine suppresses prolactin secretion. Medications which block dopamine receptors may cause a rise in prolactin levels.

Inflammatory diseases interfering with the infundibulum (hypothalamic-pituitary region) — such as sarcoidosis and histiocytosis X (unifocal and multifocal eosinophilic granuloma) may produce lesions which presumably decrease P.I.H. secretion.

Growth hormone — The stimuli which increase prolactin secretion, lower growth hormone release and, conversely, those processes which suppress prolactin increase growth hormone secretion. Hyperprolactinemia is present in approximately 30 percent of acromegalic patients.

Hypothyroidism is associated with elevated prolactin levels and, at times, with galactorrhea due to increased production of thyrotropin releasing hormone. TRH probably stimulates prolactin secretion as well as TSH production.

Puerperum (post-partum) — Prolactin, progesterone and suppressed levels of estrogen are the important prerequisites to normal post-partum milk secretion. The withdrawal of placental estrogens after delivery allows for normal lactation; this also explains why lactation does not occur during pregnancy.

Renal failure — Chronic renal failure has been associated with hyperprolactinemia.

Oral contraceptives (post-pill) — After discontinuation of birth control pills, women may experience amenorrhea. In these patients, high prolactin levels with or without galactorrhea may exist and a few may subsequently develop pituitary adenomas. A related class of medications which may lead to elevated serum prolactin is the corticosteroids.

Liver disease — Chronic liver disease may give rise to gynecomastia in men and galactorrhea in women.

Adenoma of the pituitary — Pituitary tumors may cause acromegaly, Cushing's disease (increased ACTH secretion) or hyperprolactinemia. Twenty five percent of pituitary tumors are non-secretory. Prolactinomas are slow growing and thus, only cause visual abnormalities and signs of other pituitary difficulties after years of mammary or gonadal dysfunction. A serum prolactin concentration above 150 ng per ml. is highly suggestive of a pituitary tumor.

Chiari-Frommel syndrome is defined as post partum galactorrhea which is accompanied by gonadal atrophy and persistent amenorrhea. This disorder probably results from an incomplete infundibular lesion with an associated fall in P.I.H. Forbes-Albright syndrome is a variant of this disease in which there has been no preceding pregnancy. **C** in this mnemonic can also stand for craniopharyngioma, a cystic suprasellar tumor which may produce elevated intracranial pressure without producing localizing neurologic signs.

Tranquilizers such as Thorazine and other phenothiazines, as well as the butyrophenone derivatives and opiates, are thought to interfere with the inhibitory hypothalamic effects on prolactin secretion.

Idiopathic — A fair number of cases of galactorrhea with mild elevations of prolactin will be of undertermined cause. Among this group, some subjects may harbor prolactin secreting micro-adenomas.

Nipple stimulation — Prolonged suckling can initiate lactation in non-pregnant or even in virgin women.

This acrostic does not include surgical or traumatic transection of the pituitary stalk.

Gynecomastia

Male breast enlargement must be distinguished from the pseudogynecomastia of obesity. In the latter situation the breast has a fatty rather than a truly glandular consistency. At the time of puberty as many as 70 per cent of males have transient gynecomastia. In adults, the prevalence is less than one per cent.

Mnemonic for the Causes of Gynecomastia:
T-H-R-U-S-T   M-I-L-K*

Tumors — Breast cancer is a rare but devastating disease in males. If the breast enlargement is unilateral, nodular, firm, or eccentric, biopsy should be done. Rarely, tumors such as carcinomas of lung, liver, pancreas, colon and stomach, secrete HCG and provoke gynecomastia. Adrenal, testicular and pituitary tumors are very rare causes of this abnormality.

Hemodialysis — In one third to one half of chronic hemodialysis cases, some degree of gynecomastia is seen. This occurrence is analogous to the gynecomastia induced by renourishment after periods of malnutrition. Breast development in these situations is due, at least in part, to restoration of gonadotropin secretion.

Reifenstein's syndrome is a form of incomplete testicular feminization characterized by hypospadias, small testes and gynecomastia. A related disorder, Gilbert-Dreyfus syndrome, reveals similar findings.

Ulcerative colitis — There have been case reports of an association between ulcerative colitis and gynecomastia. Some of these may have had breast development on the basis of renourishment following malnutrition and a coincidental occurrence cannot be excluded.

Spinal cord lesions — Gynecomastia has been described in patients following spinal cord trauma or in those who have sustained injury to the intercostal nerves. Of related interest is the known association between herpes zoster infection of the intercostal nerves and gynecomastia-galactorrhea.

Thyrotoxicosis — Hyperthyroidism is occasionally accompanied by gynecomastia most often in patients affected with toxic diffuse goiter. In this disorder there is increased peripheral conversion of androgens into estrogens. Sometimes gynecomastia ensues only after remission or treatment of hyperthyroidism. There may be a connection between this and the breast enlargement seen after recovery from starvation.

__M__edications make up one of the most common etiologies for breast enlargement. Estrogens used therapeutically for prostatic cancer almost always cause this finding. Androgens also cause gynecomastia due to their conversion into estrogens. Other drugs implicated include spironolactone, digoxin, reserpine, methyldopa, phenothiazines, amphetamines, imipramine, phenytoin, heroin, marijuana, cimetidine and isoniazid.

__I__diopathic (or alternatively __I__nherited) — The familial forms of gynecomastia may be inherited through an autosomal recessive or autosomal dominant gene.

__L__iver disease (chronic) — In cirrhosis, the hepatic route of estrogen inactivation is deranged. Circulating estrogen is increased, provoking dysfunctional bleeding in women and feminization in the male.

__K__linefelter's syndrome is characterized by eunuchoidism, gynecomastia and decreased testicular size. Many patients with this spectrum of findings possess an extra sex chromosome; 2 X chromosomes and 1 Y chromosome. Associated findings may include mental retardation and behavioral abnormalities; in particular, gregariousness with little substance to the content of the talk.

Secondary amenorrhea

"For a man to pretend to understand women is bad manners; for him really to understand them is bad morals."

Henry James

Secondary amenorrhea is defined as cessation of menses for more than 6 months. Essentials of history taking include a careful menstrual history and an inquiry into prior pregnancies, emotional problems, diet, medications, and sexual activity. The presence of the associated symptoms of pregnancy, thyroid disease or adrenal dysfunction must be ascertained, as well as any history of breast discharge or changes in hair distribution.

Acrostic for the Causes of Secondary Amenorrhea:
M-E-N,　O-H　P-A-U-S-E*

Medication — Approximately one percent of women who discontinue oral contraceptives after long term use will experience amenorrhea. Almost all of these patients will resume normal ovulatory periods within 6 months time. Other drugs associated with secondary amenorrhea include oral steroid preparations, phenothiazines, haloperidol, imipramine, spironolactone, methyldopa and cyclophosphamide.

Expectancy — Pregnancy is the most frequent cause of secondary amennorrhea and excluding its presence is the initial part of the evaluation of this clinical problem. An HCG precipitation slide test performed 6 weeks after the last menstrul period has a sensitivity greater than 90 percent. If a high index of suspicion remains, in spite of a negative test, the clinician can either repeat the test in one week or obtain a serum HCG beta subunit determination.

Nutritional abnormalities — Crash dieting, sudden weight loss and anorexia nervosa can trigger alterations in the hypothalamic pituitary axis. At the opposite end of the spectrum, marked obesity has also been associated with secondary amenorrhea.

Ovarian dysfunction — Ovarian failure may occur physiologically as in normal menopause or may be the result of iatrogenic causes such as radiation therapy or chemotherapy. In these instances, determination of serum gonadotropins will reveal elevated FSH and LH. Bilateral ovarian neoplasms are rare causes of ovarian failure, although granulosa cell tumors and arrhenoblastomas may produce excessive steroids, thus causing amenorrhea. In Stein-Leventhal syndrome, continual LH secretion is probably responsible for the amenorrhea, infertility, hirsutism and enlarged polycystic ovaries seen in this disorder.

Hypothyroidism (and **H**yperthyroidism) may be accompanied by amenorrhea. Mild hypothyroidism is a cause of hyperprolactinemia and, by this mechanism, may cause galactorrhea as well as cessation of menses. In hyperthyroidism, oligomenorrhea and amenorrhea occur more frequently than menorrhagia.

Pituitary tumors are capable of destroying pituitary tissue or may stimulate prolactin secretion. In the former instance gonadotropin levels tend to be low. In the latter situation prolactin levels are elevated. About 30 percent of those patients with amenorrhea and hyperprolactinemia will have detectable tumors by computerized axial tomography.

Adrenal hyperfunction — In Cushing's syndrome, amenorrhea is frequently present along with other signs of glucocorticoid excess such as weight gain, weakness, impaired glucose tolerance, hirsutism and hypertension.

Uterine causes — Radiation therapy, endometrial curettage or septic abortion can lead to adhesions and obliteration of the uterine cavity (Asherman's syndrome). Trauma to the cervical os can, likewise, cause scarring and obstruction of menstrual flow.

Systemic disease (such as malignancy, collagen vascular diseases, acute or chronic infections and poorly controlled diabetes mellitus).

Emotional stress can trigger changes in the normal functioning of the hypothalamic-pituitary axis. FSH and estrogen stimulation in this form of functional amenorrhea generally remain normal. However, cyclic LH secretion is absent and, under prolonged stress, this lack of LH release may eventually become permanent.

Signs of Belladonna Poisoning

The Renaissance women of Italy used an extract of the deadly nightshade to provoke pupillary mydriasis in order to improve their appearance. Thus, the extract obtained the name "belladonna," meaning beautiful woman in Italian, but in English meaning terrible poison. Obviously nothing was lost in the translation.

Following is a well-known verse for recalling the signs of belladonna poisoning:

Hot as a Hare	(Temperature elevation and rapid pulse)
Mad as a Hen	(Restless, confused, and occasionally with delirium and psychosis)
Blind as a Bat	(Blurred vision, photophobia, dilated pupils)
Red as a Beet	(Flushed skin)
Dry as a Bone	(Dry mouth and skin, difficulty swallowing)

Other manifestations of parasympathetic blockade not included in this list are urinary retention and abdominal distention.

Venereal Diseases

In 1492, while Columbus was exporting diseases to the Americas, Heironymus Fracastorius was composing a Latin poem describing the scourges accompanying the armies which ravaged (and ravished) Italy. The main character of the epic poem was a swine herd named Syphilis (pig-lover). Short-sighted Syphilis made the egregious error of offering sacrifice to the local king rather than to the more powerful sun god. For this, Syphilis was cursed with a venereal disease; his one little 'boo boo' led to many more buboes.

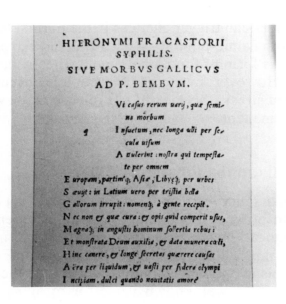

The title page to the original edition of Fracastorius's poem about Syphilis the swineherd

196

An Acrostic for Recalling the List of Sexually Transmitted Diseases:

C-H-A-N-C-Re-S = G-U-I-L-T*

Chlamydia — Chlamydia trachomatis is the main causative organism of nongonococcal urethritis. In men under the age of 35 it is a prevalent cause of epididymitis. It is also more frequently being recognized as a cause of pelvic inflammatory disease in women. A chlamydial organism is also responsible for lymphogranuloma venereum.

Herpes — After an incubation period of approximately 4 days, the primary vesicular lesions erupt on the genitalia, ulcerate and eventually dry and crust. Eighty per cent of primary infections are type 2 herpes genitalis and an even greater number of recurrent infections are type 2. The average duration of primary infections is 3 weeks, but is only about 12 days for recurrences. Virus shedding occurs mainly within the first 5 days of infection.

Amebiasis is one etiology of the gay-bowel syndrome.

Neisseria gonorrhea — In the male, dysuria and a urethral discharge usually occurs 3 to 5 days after exposure, although up to 10 percent of infected males may be asymptomatic. The gram stain of the discharge reveals pairs of gram-negative intracellular cocci and is diagnostic in the male patient. Diagnosis in the female must be made from cervical cultures on Thayer-Martin medium. Ten to 17 percent of affected women will develop P.I.D.

Condyloma acuminata are venereal warts; painless papillomas affecting the genital and perianal area.

Reiter's syndrome is not an infectious cause of urethritis but symptoms may be perpetuated by continued sexual contact. Other manifestations include conjunctivitis, keratoderma blennorrhagica, and polyarthritis. (see the acrostic G-R-A-S-P p. 138).

Syphilis — The course of syphilis may be divided into several phases: primary, secondary, latent and tertiary. Primary syphilis is manifest as the genital chancre, although depending on sexual practices it may also arise in the anal canal, oral mucosa or on the hands. Secondary syphilis may reveal itself as a flu-like illness with lymphadenopathy. A generalized skin eruption is also characteristic. Ten to 40 years after the primary infection, one third of untreated individuals develop tertiary syphilis which can take several forms; cardiovascular syphilis, neurosyphilis or isolated gummas.

Granuloma inguinale is caused by the gram-negative bacterium Donovania granulomatis. Painless slow growing genital ulcers are characteristic. In men, lesions are usually located on the glans, prepuce or shaft of the penis. In women, the labia are the most frequently affected site.

Ureaplasma urealyticum is a form of mycoplasma which is responsible for a small percentage of cases of nongonococcal urethritis. As with chlamydia trachomatis, patients generally have a longer symptomatic period than that of gonorrhea (2 to 4 days in gonorrhea) and a less purulent discharge.

Infectious hepatitis — Hepatitis B surface antigen has been measured in blood, saliva, breast milk, tears, synovial fluid,

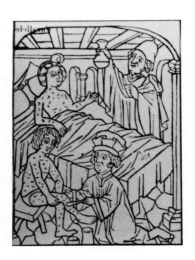

Picture from a pamphlet used to educate the public about syphilis. (From the year 1497)

198

intestinal fluid, urine, and seminal fluid. High attack rates occur in sexual partners, especially in the homosexual population.

Lice (and scabies) — are passed by intimate contact and present with pubic pruritis. The latter infestation, caused by mites, produces burrows which should be scraped and examined microscopically. Lice or "crabs" may be seen with the naked eye.

Trichomonas causes a vaginitis which may be perpetuated by continued sexual contact. Wet mount of the vaginal discharge will demonstrate the motile, flagellated parasite.

Notable exclusions from this list are chancroid, and hemophilus vaginalis.

Genital Ulcers

When confronted by the patient with genital ulcers, the clinician should place special emphasis on examination of the skin, eyes, oral mucosa, joints, inguinal lymph nodes, anus and rectum. Swabbing for cultures and scrapings for microscopic examination, including Gram stains, should be performed. It is prudent to recall that frequently more than one venereal infection resides in the same patient.

Acrostic for the Causes of Genital Ulcers:
B-I-G   C-H-A-N-C-R-E-S*

Behcet's syndrome — In this rare disorder, oral and genital ulcers may be accompanied by uveitis and central nervous system involvement. The ulcers may occur on the vulva, scrotum or penis; they are deep, well circumscribed and heal with scarring.

Injury — e.g. bites, zipper accidents, and oral sexual activity among people with dental braces.

Granuloma inguinale is caused by the gram-negative, encapsulated bacterium, Donovania granulomatis. It is rarely seen in temperate climates. The genital lesion starts as a painless macule, develops into a papule, and erodes into an erythematous granuloma. The ulcer first affects the glans penis or vulva and then spreads to the penile shaft or vagina and perianal area.

Chancroid is widespread in parts of Africa and Asia, but is infrequent in the United States. It is caused by the gram-negative bacillus, Hemophilus ducreyi which produces a pustule that erodes into a shallow, ragged and painful ulcer. The margins are red and a gray foul-smelling exudate is often present along with painful unilateral bubos.

Herpes — In genital herpes, grouped vesicles on erythematous bases are noted on the glans and shaft in the male and on the labia mucosa and surrounding skin in the female. The vesicles break, creating painful shallow ulcers. Giant cells and inclusion bodies on a scraping of these lesions is strongly suggestive of the diagnosis.

Antibiotic — Tetracycline may cause a fixed drug eruption consisting of red plaques and ulcers on the glans penis.

iNsect — (mite bite) Scabies causes pruritic papules in the genital area, popliteal fossae, around the waist and between the fingers and hands. The infesting mite, Sarcoptes scabiei, has eight legs, transverse corrugations and hair like projections on its dorsal body. The female mite burrows 2 mm into the stratum corneum each day, laying eggs on her route and dying after 1 to 2 months.

Carcinoma — An ulcer which remains undiagnosed or does not respond to therapeutic maneuvers should alert the physician to the possibility of carcinoma.

Reiter's syndrome may be precipitated by many factors such as salmonella, yersinia or shigella gastroenteritis, or by venereal contact. Recurrent attacks are common and may present as painless, erosive and exudative lesions on the scrotum or penis. Balanitis circinata, superficial reddened erosions which completely circumscribe the glans, occurs frequently.

Erythroplasia of Queyrat is related to Bowens disease, a chronic, slowly-growing squamous cell epithelioma. Well-demarcated, erythematous, velvety patches are found on the glans, the prepuce or the vulva. Regional lymph nodes may reveal metastatic disease. In particular, the patient should be questioned about a history of arsenic contact.

<u>S</u>yphilis — The first manifestation of primary syphilis, the chancre, appears 3 to 4 weeks after infection at any site where the treponemes have entered the body. It usually begins as a flat, indurated papular lesion and evolves into a smooth, clean, and painless erosion which exudes serous fluid. A single, nontender, enlarged regional lymph node is often present. Darkfield microscopy is the most reliable method of early diagnosis, but is not useful with oral lesions because of the presence of other normally occurring treponemes.

False Positive VDRL Tests for Syphilis

The VDRL slide flocculation test is a means of quantitating the nonspecific reagin antibody noted in syphilis. It is positive in 70 percent of cases of primary syphilis, 100 percent of cases of secondary syphilis, and 70 percent of those patients with latent or late syphilis. It has been estimated that approximately one third of positive reagin test are false positives. In these, the VDRL titers do not exceed 1:8.

The more specific treponemal antibody test the FTA-ABS test, is very specific and is used for confirmation of a positive VDRL. A false positive FTA-ABS occasionally occurs in pregnancy and in individuals with S.L.E. The FTA-ABS should routinely be performed in those patients with negative VDRL'S, suspected of having late, latent or primary syphilis. Recall the rhyme:

> With the VDRL
> You can never tell,
> But the FTA
> Never goes away.*

Mnemonic for False Positive VDRL'S:

V-D-R-L-S	,V-D-R-L-S*
Vaccination — smallpox.	**V**iral infection — acute viral infections, especially infectious mononucleosis, (also bacterial infections, mycoplasma, malaria)
Drug addiction — (heroin) 25 percent of narcotic addicts have false positive VDRL's.	**D**rug — e.g. hydralazine, and other medications which may cause drug-induced lupus.
Rheumatoid arthritis — In 15 to 45 percent of chronic false positive reactors there is an associated collagen vascular disorder.	**R**heumatic fever
Lupus — Chronic biological false positive VDRL'S in SLE are associated with circulating anticoagulants.	**L**eprosy
Senescience — Approximately 10 per cent of patients over the age of 70 will have false positive reagin tests for syphilis.	**S**ubacute bacterial endocarditis

The main causes of false positive VDRL'S can also be recalled by remembering four words beginning with **A**:

> **A**ge (old age)
> **A**ddict
> **A**ntibody proliferation
> **A**cute infection*

Causes of Cataracts

Opacifications of the lens or its capsule are extremely common in the adult population. Many cataracts, however, do not progress to obstruct vision. When they do, the patient may complain of seeing halos around lights, difficulty with night driving or changes in the appearance of colors, particularly blue and yellow. The individual with central lens opacities may actually notice improved visual acuity in dimmer light when mydriasis compensates for the blocking effect of the cataract.

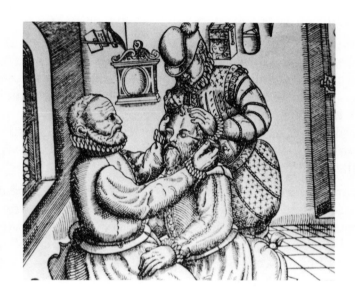

A 15th century Dutch print demonstrating a cataract extraction

Mnemonic for the Causes of Cataract Formation:
How-D-I-M   ,   So-D-I-M*

<u>H</u>ow — **H**ypoparathyroidism may be postoperative, idiopathic or familial and presents many symptoms and signs which start with letter **C**; Calcium concentration lowered, cutaneous calcification, cramps, carpopedal spasm, Chvostek's sign, convulsions, cardiac arrythmnias, CNS calcification (basal

ganglia), candidiasis (familial form) and cataracts (due to lowered calcium levels in the aqueous humor).

Diabetes — The cataracts seen in diabetics are usually of the senile variety, although they occur earlier in life and progress more rapidly. Another more specific type of cataract occurs in young diabetics and characteristically develops under the anterior and posterior lens capsules as a network of white snowflake-like flecks. Sustained hyperglycemia and subsequent sorbitol accumulation in the lens fibers both play a role in the development of diabetic cataracts.

Infection or **I**njury — Chronic infection, intraocular foreign bodies, blunt or penetrating ocular trauma, radiation injury.

Myotonic dystrophy is a hereditary disorder featuring myotonia (an inability to relax a muscle normally after contraction), an expressionless face with associated ptosis, muscular atrophy, frontal alopecia, testicular atrophy, and cataracts. The lens opacities, revealed in slit lamp examination, are fine, scintillating subcapsular deposits virtually diagnostic of the disorder. Blepharoconjunctivitis is a commonly associated ocular finding.

So — **S**enile cataracts are, by far, the most frequent type of cataract seen and are of two varieties. The nuclear type which begins soon after the age of 40, is very slow growing, and develops out of the nucleus of the lens. The cortical cataract is peripheral, wedge shaped, and progresses more rapidly than the nuclear form.

Drugs — Drugs reported to induce cataract formation include ergot, dinitrophenol, naphthalene, phenothiazines, and triparanol. Individuals on long term corticosteroid therapy may develop posterior subcapsular cataracts.

Idiopathic — This group includes hereditary cataracts and cataracts in childhood associated with a host of metabolic disturbances and systemic disorders.

Mongolism — Down's syndrome and other chromosomal aberrations, including Turner's syndrome, are disorders in which cataracts are prone to develop. Other ocular findings in Down's syndrome include the presence of a medial epican-

thal fold and Brushfield's spots, gray-white areas of depigmentation in the iris.

Orthostatic Hypotension; A Song
Music and Lyric by Robert L. Bloomfield/©1982 J. Herring, R.
Bloomfield

The musical manuscript format had to be deleted to make
room for the explanatory material in the margin.

	LYRICS	NOTES
Verse 1:	When I cough	Tussive syncope — after a paroxysm of coughing usually in people with chronic bronchitis.
	When I swallow	Glossopharyngeal reflex syncope.
	When air distends a viscus which is hollow	Pain initiates a vaso-vagal reflex.
	Shy-Drager, Riley-Day, Holmes-Adie, don't forget Guillain-Barre.	Primary autonomic insufficiency syndromes. Acute idiopathic polyneuritis often preceded by viral infection.
	With Parkinson's, and Addison's	Hypovolemia
	At times with carcinoid when I flush, or push too much, and sometimes when I void.	Vasodilation due to circulating bradykinin, heat or catecholamines. Valsalva decreased venous return. Micturation syncope is seen in elderly during or after urination. Vasomotor reflexes play a role.

Chorus: (Sung by patient)	I'm falling for you, what are you gonna do? Don't tell me just to take my time And get up nice and slow.	
	I will pay your fee, But not just for your sympathy, What's wrong with me I really want to know.	
Verse 2:	Pheochroma —cytoma	Paroxysmal hypertension only occurs in 50 percent. Postural hypotension does occur.
	Acute glaucoma	Related to pain and vasovagal reflex.
	Atrial myxoma	Decreased cardiac output (rare tumor).
	Both forms of diabetes	Diabetes mellitus — peripheral neuropathic changes affects vasculature. Diabetes insipidus-hypovolemia.
	Too much Reunite	Alcohol related causes — depressed reflexes, hypovolemia, hypoglycemia.
	Not eating your Wheaties.	Deconditioning, e.g. prolonged bed rest.
	Parasympathetic flow or paraneoplastic.	Usually solid tumors.
	Pregnancy and	Peripheral vasodilation and increased placental flow.

plasma loss,	e.g. dehydration or exsanguination.
When veins lost their elastic.	Varicosities
(Repeat Chorus)	

Verse 3:	Nitrates,	Venodilatation and arteriolar dilation.
	Diuretics,	Decreased plasma volume.
	Narcotics,	Also other medications such as antihypertensives.
	Let's hope I'm not tabetic.	Tabes dorsalis.
	My carotid won't behave	Carotid sinus sensitivity may be initiated . . .
	It acts up everytime I try to shave.	by turning head, tight collars, or by shaving.
	Uremia, anemia M.I or T.I.A.	Decreased cardiac output or cerebral ischemia.
	Cord lesions above T_6	Loss of sympathetic tone.
	Please check my serum K +.	Hypokalemia.
Chorus:	I'm falling for you, What are you gonna do? Don't tell me just to take my time And get up nice and slow. I will pay the fee, But it's not my sympathectomy,	

Is my pulse of 44 too slow?
Just how low can my blood pressure go, oh!
What's wrong with me I really want to know, — ow, — ow.*

e.g. Bradyarrhythmias
Stokes-Adams attacks.

(A harmonious rendition of this song on cassette tape can be obtained by sending $2.75 to Harbinger Press, Box 17201, Winston-Salem, N.C. 27106. Make check payable to R.L. Bloomfield).

INVITATION TO OUR READERS

Do you know an unusual mnemonic? If so, please send it to us with the source of its origin. If we don't already have it and if we print it in a subsequent book, we will send you a free copy of the book and, of course, give you credit. Thank you all.

Write: Harbinger Press, P.O. Box 17201
Winston-Salem, N.C. 27106

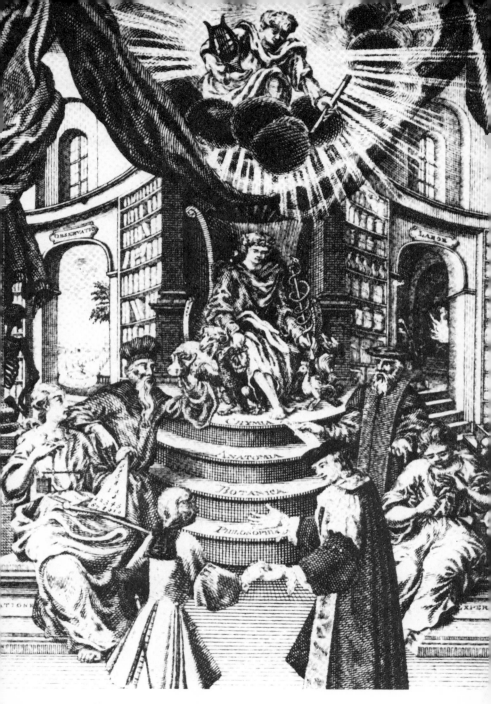

The frontispiece from Herman Boerhaave's book on concise maxims.

The wrangling and unseemly disputes which have often disgraced our profession arise, in a great majority of cases, on the one hand, from this morbid sensitiveness to the confession of error and on the other, from a lack of brotherly consideration and a convenient forgetfulness of our own failings.

Osler
Teacher & Student 1892

The greatest discoveries of surgery are anesthesia, asepsis and roentgenology and none was discovered by a surgeon.

Martin Henry Fischer

Spinal Motor and Sensory Levels in Spinal Cord Injuries

I Motor

Spinal Cord Level	Impaired Movement (and muscles involved)
C_2, C_3	Breathing (Diaphragm),
C_4, C_5	Shoulder Shrugging (trapezius)
C_5, C_6	Flexion of forearm (Biceps, Brachealis)
C_6, C_7	Extension at wrist (Extensor/carpi radialis longus and brevis)
C_7, C_8	Extension of arm at elbow (triceps)
C_8, T_1	Finger abduction and adduction (Interossei and Lumbricals)
L_1, L_2, L_3	Hip flexion and adduction (Iliopsoas, Adductor longus and brevis)
L_2, L_3, L_4	Knee extension and ankle dorsiflexion (Quadriceps and tibialis anterior)
L_5, S_1	Extension of great toe (Extensor hallucis longus)
S_1, S_2	Ankle plantarflexion (Gastrocnemius, Soleus)
S_2, S_3, S_4	Anal sphincter contraction (Sphincter ani externus)

II Sensory

Spinal Cord Level	Border of Sensory Deficit
$C_2 - C_4$	Neck and clavicle
C_5	Outer deltoid
C_6	Thumb
C_7	Middle finger
C_8	Little finger
T_1	Medial arm
T_{3-4}	Nipple
T_{10}	Umbilicus
L_1	Inguinal region
L_3	Medial knee
L_4	Medial ankle, Great toe
L_5	Dorsum of foot
S_1	Lateral foot and small toe
$S_3 - S_5$	Perianal area

Helpful Features in Distinguishing Between:

Glomerulonephritis and	Interstitial Nephritis
Proteinuria usually greater than 3 grm/24 hr.	Proteinuria less than 1.5 grm/24 hr.
Sodium handling normal until late in disease	Sodium wasting in urine
Uric acid slightly elevated	Uric acid markedly elevated
Anemia present	Anemia severe for degree of renal insufficiency
Acidosis tends to be normochloremic	Hyperchloremic acidosis
Hypertension common	Hypertension may or may not be present
Sediment shows numerous cells and casts	Urine sediment shows few cells and few casts

Causes of Renal Tubular Acidosis

Type I (Distal)	Type II (Proximal)
Sjogren's syndrome	Amyloidosis
Lupus erythematosus	Fanconi's syndrome
Medullary sponge kidney	Medullary cystic disease
Cirrhosis	Nephrotic syndrome
Renal transplantation	Renal transplantation
Inherited	Inherited
Amphotericin B	Outdated tetracycline
Toluene intoxication	Cadmium poisoning

Immune Complex Diseases

Serum sickness (drugs, antisera)
Systemic Lupus Erythematosus
Rheumatoid Arthritis
Poststreptococcal glomerulonephritis
Hypersensitivity pneumonitis
Mixed cryoglobulinemia
Bacterial endocarditis
Viral infections — hepatitis B, infectious mononucleosis
Polyarteritis

Features Suggesting Benign vs Malignant Disease in Solitary Pulmonary Nodules

Benign	Malignant
Doubling time — Inflammatory lesions double in volume in less than 5 weeks	Malignant lesions generally take 1 to 18 months to double in size
Benign nodules take longer than 18 months. No change in 2 years — probably benign.	
Age less than 30 — probability of malignancy less than 2 per cent	Older patient — Risk increased by about 15 per cent for each decade over 30 50-59; 41% 60-69; 50% 70-79; 70% over 80 almost 100%
Central core calcification, lamination or dense generalized calcification suggests a benign lesion	may calcify

Differentiating Features of Hemoptysis vs. Hematemesis

Hemoptysis	Hematemesis
Blood is coughed up	Blood is vomited
Usually frothy	Never frothy
Usually bright red	Dark red
Alkaline	Acid
Preceded by a gurgling sound	Usually preceded by nausea
Blood-tinged sputum lasts several days	Blood-tinged sputum absent
Contains pus, organisms or macrophages	May contain food particles
Anemia may or may not be present	Often anemic before actual hematemesis

Vertigo: Peripheral vs. Central Origin

Peripheral	Central
Acute onset	Gradual onset
Paroxysmal	Usually continuous
Severe	Usually mild
Lasts minutes to hours occasionally days	Days to months or even years
Positional nystagmus is consistent in all fields of gaze	Nystagmus changes in different fields of gaze
Head position markedly affects vertigo	Head position has slight or no influence on vertigo
Fatiguable — nystagmus and vertigo subside after repetitive testing	Nonfatiguable
Tinnitus and hearing loss common	Rare
Cranial nerve abnormalities rare	Cranial nerve dysfunction common

Diagnostic Criteria for Rheumatoid Arthritis

A. *Classical Rheumatoid Arthritis*

This diagnosis requires seven of the following criteria. In criteria 1 through 5 the joint signs or symptoms must be continuous for at least six weeks. (Any one of the features listed under "Exclusions" will exclude a patient from this and all other categories).

1. Morning stiffness.
2. Pain on motion or tenderness in at least one joint (observed by a physician).
3. Swelling (soft tissue thickening or fluid, not bony overgrowth alone) in at least one joint (observed by a physician).
4. Swelling (observed by a physician) of at least one other joint (any interval free of joint symptoms between the two joint involvements may not be more than 3 months).
5. Symmetrical joint swelling (observed by a physician) with simultaneous involvement of the same joint on both sides of the body (bi-lateral involvement of proximal interphalangeal, metacarpophalangeal, or metatarsophalangeal joints is acceptable without absolute symmetry). Terminal phalangeal joint involvement will not satisfy this criterion.
6. Subcutaneous nodules (observed by a physican) over bony prominences, or extensor surfaces or in juxta-articular regions.
7. Roentgenographic changes typical of rheumatoid arthritis (which must include at least bony decalcification localized to or most marked adjacent to the involved joints and not just degenerative changes). Degenerative changes do not exclude patients from any group classified as rheumatoid arthritis.
8. Positive agglutination test — demonstration of the "rheumatoid factor" by any method which, in two laboratories, has been positive in not over 5% of normal controls — or positive streptococcal agglutination test. [The latter is now obsolete.]
9. Poor mucin precipitate from synovial fluid (with shreds and cloudy solution).
10. Characteristic histologic changes in synovium with three or more of the following: marked villous hypertrophy; proliferation of superficial synovial cells often with palisading; marked infiltration of chronic inflammatory cells (lymphocytes or plasma cells predominating) with tendency to form "lymphoid nodules"; deposition of compact fibrin either on surface or intersitially; foci or necrosis.
11. Characteristic histologic changes in nodules showing granulomatous foci with central zones of cell necrosis, surrounded by a palisade of proliferated macrophages, and peripheral fibrosis and chronic inflammatory cell infiltration, predominantly perivascular.

B. *Definite Rheumatoid Arthritis*

This diagnosis requires five of the above criteria. In criteria 1 through 5 the joint signs or symptoms must be continuous for at least six weeks.

C. *Probable Rheumatoid Arthritis*

This diagnosis requires three of the above criteria. In at least one of criteria 1 through 5 the joint signs or symptoms must be continuous for at least six weeks.

D. *Possible Rheumatoid Arthritis*

This diagnosis requires two of the following criteria and total duration of joint symptoms must be at least three weeks.

1. Morning stiffness.
2. Tenderness or pain on motion (observed by a physician) with history of recurrence or persistence for three weeks.
3. History or observation of joint swelling.
4. Subcutaneous nodules (observed by a physician).
5. Elevated sedimentation rate or C-reactive protein.
6. Iritis [of dubious value as a criterion except in the case of juvenile rheumatoid arthritis.]

E. *Exclusions*

1. The typical rash of *systemic lupus erythematosus* (with butterfly distribution, follicle plugging, and areas of atrophy).
2. High concentration of *Lupus erythematosus* cells (four or more in two smears prepared from

heparinized blood incubated not over two hours) [or other clearcut evidence of systemic lupus erythematosus.]

3. Histologic evidence of *periarteritis nodosa* with segmental necrosis of arteries associated with nodular leukocytic infiltration extending perivascularly and tending to include many eosinophils.

4. Weakness of neck, trunk, and pharyngeal muscles or persistent muscle swelling or *dermatomyositis*.

5. Definite *scleroderma* (not limited to the fingers). [The latter is an arguable point.]

6. A clinical picture characteristic of *rheumatic fever* with migratory joint involvement and evidence of endocarditis, especially if accompanied by subcutaneous nodules or erythema marginatum or chorea. (An elevated antistreptolysin titer will not rule out the diagnosis of rheumatoid arthritis).

7. A clinical picture characteristic of *gouty arthritis* with acute attacks of swelling, redness, and pain in one or more joints, especially if relieved by colchicine.

8. Tophi.

9. A clinical picture characteristic of acute *infectious arthritis* of bacterial or viral origin with: an acute focus of infection or in close association with a disease of known infectious origin; chills; fever; and an acute joint involvement, usually migratory initially (especially if there are organisms in the joint fluid or response to antibiotic therapy).

10. *Tubercule bacilli* in the joints or histological evidence of joint tuberculosis.

11. A clinical picture characteristic of *Reiter's syndrome* with urethritis and conjunctivitis associated with acute joint involvement, usually migratory initially.

12. A clinical picture characteristic of the *shoulder-hand syndrome* with unilateral involvement of shoulder and hand, with diffuse swelling of the hand followed by atrophy and contractures.

13. A clinical picture characteristic of *hypertrophic osteoarthropathy* with clubbing of fingers and/or hypertrophic periostitis along the shafts of the long bones especially if an intrapulmonary lesion (or other appropriate underlying disorder) is present.,

14. A clinical picture characteristic of *neuroarthropathy* with condensation and destruction of bones of involved joints and with associated neurologic findings.

15. *Homogentisic acid* in the urine, detectable grossly with alkalinization.

16. Histologic evidence of *sarcoid* or positive Kveim test.

17. *Multiple myeloma* as evidenced by marked increase in plasma cells in the bone marrow, or Bence-Jones protein in the urine.

18. Characteristic skin lesions of *erythema nodosum*.

19. *Leukemia* or *lymphoma* with characteristic cells in peripheral blood, bone marrow or tissue.

20. *Agammaglobulinemia*.

These criteria were developed prior to the new classification of rheumatic diseases adopted by the American Rheumatism Association in which ankylosing spondylitis, psoriatic arthritis, and arthritis associated with ulcerative colitis and regional enteritis are listed as distinct from rheumatoid arthritis.

The definitive diagnosis of adrenal hypofuntion can be done with ACTH stimulation tests:

A) Outpatient screening:

    1. Obtain baseline blood cortisol and aldosterone levels.

    2. Administer I.M. 25 units (0.25mg) of alpha 1-24 corticotropin.

    3. Measure blood cortisol and aldosterone levels 30 and 60 minutes afterward.

    4. In normal subjects: blood cortisol levels often double and rise 7-10 micrograms per 100 ml over the control values and

aldosterone increases 5-15 nanograms per 100 ml above the initial values.

B) Intravenous ACTH testing of adrenal reserve:

    1) Minimize danger of acute adrenal crisis provoked by testing by prior administration of 1 mg dexamethasone.

2) Use normal saline I.V. set-up.
3) Infuse 40 units of ACTH or 25 units of alpha 1-24 corticoprin daily over eight hours for 4-5 days.
4) Collect 24-hour urines daily and test for creatinine, 17-hydroxycorticoid and 17 ketosteroid levels.
5) Patients with primary adrenal insufficiency will demonstrate a rise of less than 2 mg per day in steroid excretion.
6) Patients with incomplete adrenal insufficiency tend to have subnormal increments in urinary 17-hydroxycorticosteroids.

Upper Limits of Normal Q-T Intervals (in seconds)

Heart Rate	Men	Women
150	0.25	0.28
136	0.26	0.29
125	0.28	0.30
115	0.39	0.32
107	0.30	0.33
100	0.31	0.34
93	0.32	0.35
88	0.33	0.36
78	0.35	0.38
75	0.36	0.39
71	0.37	0.40
68	0.38	0.41
65	0.38	0.42
62	0.39	0.43
60	0.40	0.44
57	0.41	0.45
55	0.42	0.46
52	0.42	0.47
51	0.43	0.47
50	0.44	0.48
48	0.45	0.49
46	0.45	0.50
45	0.46	0.51

Date 1300 B.C.

Name Mr. Schlamazzel   D.O.B. _____

Address _____

Rx

ABRACADABRA

60

Repeat twice t.i.d.
until gone

☐ Refill (NR) 1 2 3 4
☐ Refill to maintain above directions one year only. Dispensing Limit. The greater of a 34 day supply or 100 unit doses.

I Dr. Ben Osler

Product Selection Permitted   Dispense as Written

216

BIBLIOGRAPHY

1. Adams R. Victor M. Principles of Neurology. New York: McGraw-Hill, 1977.
2. Altschule M. What Medicine is About. Boston: The Francis A. Countway Library of Medicine, 1975.
3. Aristides N. Dismembrances of Things Present. The American Scholar, Spring 1980: 157-164.
4. Bean W., ed. Aphorisms from Latham. Iowa City: Prairie Press, 1962.
5. Bettmann O. A Pictorial History of Medicine. Springfield: Charles C. Thomas, 1956.
6. Beveridge W. The Art of Scientific Investigation. New York: W.W. Norton and Company, Inc., 1957.
7. Birnholz J. Michelson P. Clinical Diagnostic Pearls. New York: Medical Examination Publishing Company, Inc., 1971.
8. Bursztayn H. Hamm R. Medical Maxims, Two Views of Science. The Yale Journal of Biology and Medicine, 52: 483-486, 1979.
9. Castiglioni A. A History of Medicine. New York: Alfred A. Knopf, 1946.
10. Center S. The Art of Book Reading. New York: Charles Scribner's Sons, 1952.
11. Cermak L. Improving Your Memory. New York: W.W. Norton and Company, 1975.
12. Church M. Don Quixote: The Knight of La Mancha. New York: New York University Press, 1971.
13. Collins D. Dynamic Differential Diagnosis. Philadelphia: Lippincott, 1981.
14. Constant J. Bedside Cardiology. 2nd ed. Boston: Little Brown and Co., 1976.
15. Coope R. The Quiet Art. Edinburgh: E. and S. Livingston, Ltd., 1958.
16. De Gowin E. DeGowin R. Bedside Diagnostic Examination. New York: MacMillan Publishing Co., Inc., 1976.
17. Done A. The Toxic Emergency. Emergency Medicine, Vol. 14, No. 1, January 15, 1982: 42-77.
18. Drachman D. The Neurobiology of Memory. Neurology Review Vol. 1181, Issue 3 October 1981.
19. Educational Development of Man. Collected Papers: Mayo Clinic Foundation Vol. 20, 1928: 937-942.
20. Eliot C. American Contributions to Civilization and Other Essays and Addresses. New York: The Century Co., 1897.
21. Fishman M. Hoffman A. Klausner R. Rockson S. Thaler M. Medicine. Philadelphia: Lippincott, 1981.
22. Gorrol A. May L. Mulley A. Primary Care Medicine. Philadelphia: Lippincott, 1981.
23. Gottleib A. Zamkoff K. Jastremski M. Scalzo A. Imboden K. The Whole Internist Catalogue. Philadelphia: W.B. Sanders, 1980.
24. Harrington J. The School of Salerno. New York: Paul B. Hoeber, 1920.
25. Harvey A. McGehee Richard J. McKusick V. Owens A. The Principles and Practice of Medicine, 20th ed. New York: Appleton-Century-Croft, 1980.
26. Holbrook J. Physical Diagnosis Review. New York: Medical Examination Publishing Company, 1979.
27. Holland J. Frei E. Cancer Medicine, 2nd ed. Philadelphia: Lea & Febiger, 1982.
28. Isselbacher K. Adams R. Braunwald R. Petersdorf R. Wilson J. Harrisons Principles of Internal Medicine, 9th ed. New York: McGraw-Hill, 1980.
29. James W. Memories and Studies. New York: Longmans Green and Co., 1934.
30. Lazarus G. Goldsmith L. Diagnosis of Skin Disease. Philadelphia: FA Davis Company, 1982.
31. Lorayne H. Lucas J. The Memory Book. New York: Ballantine Books, 1974.
32. McCarty Daniel J. Arthritis and Allied Conditions, 9th ed. Philadelphia: Lea & Febiger, 1979.
33. Miller J. The Body In Question. New York: Random House, 1978.
34. Montgomery R. Memory Made Easy. New York: AMACOM, 1979.

35. Nelson G. How to See. Boston: Little Brown and Company, 1977.
36. Osler W. Aequanimitas With Other Addresses, 3rd ed. Philadelphia: The Blakiston Company, 1932.
37. Prager S. Barza M. Diagnostic Imperatives. New York: Thieme-Stratton Inc., 1981.
38. Santayana G. Interpretation of Poetry and Religion. New York: C. Scribner's Sons, 1900.
39. Scheie H. Daniel M. Textbook of Ophthalmology, 9th ed. Philadelphia: W.B. Saunders Company, 1977.
40. Schouten J. The Rod and Serpent of Asklepios. Amsterdam: Elsevier Publishing Company, 1967.
41. Schrier, R., ed. Renal and Electrolyte Disorders. Boston: Little Brown and Company, 1976.
42. Sire J. How to Read Slowly. Downer's Grove, Ill: Inter Varsity Press, 1978.
43. Spiro H. Clinical Gastroenterology. New York: MacMillan Publishing Company, 1977.
44. Spivak, J. Barnes H. Manual of Clinical Problems in Internal Medicine, 2nd ed. Boston: Little Brown and Company, 1978.
45. Starrett V. The Private Life of Sherlock Holmes. Chicago: The University of Chicago Press, 1960.
46. Strauss M., ed., Familiar Medical Quotations. Boston: Little Brown and Company, 1968.
47. Toffler A. Future Shock. New York: Bantam, 1971.
48. Williams W. Hematology. New York: McGraw-Hill, 1977.
49. Yates F. The Art of Memory. Chicago: The University of Chicago Press, 1966.

219

220

221

222